LARYNGEAL CANCER
An Interdisciplinary Resource for Practitioners

LARYNGEAL CANCER
An Interdisciplinary Resource for Practitioners

Editors

Jennifer Campion Friberg, EdD, CCC-SLP/L, ASHA Fellow
Cross Endowed Chair in the Scholarship of Teaching and Learning
Associate Professor
Department of Communication Sciences and Disorders
Illinois State University
Normal, Illinois

Lisa A. Vinney, PhD, CCC-SLP/L
Assistant Professor
Department of Communication Sciences and Disorders
Illinois State University
Normal, Illinois

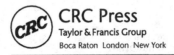

CRC Press
Taylor & Francis Group
Boca Raton London New York

CRC Press is an imprint of the
Taylor & Francis Group, an **informa** business

Laryngeal Cancer: An Interdisciplinary Resource for Practitioners, includes ancillary materials specifically available for faculty use. Included are PowerPoint Slides. Please visit http://www.routledge.com/9781630911591 to obtain access.

First published 2017 by SLACK Incorporated

Published 2024 by CRC Press
2385 NW Executive Center Drive, Suite 320, Boca Raton FL 33431

and by CRC Press
4 Park Square, Milton Park, Abingdon, Oxon, OX14 4RN

CRC Press is an imprint of Taylor & Francis Group, LLC

© 2017 Taylor & Francis Group, LLC

Cover photo reprinted with permission of Molly Friberg.

Library of Congress Cataloging-in-Publication Data

Names: Friberg, Jennifer C., 1974- editor. | Vinney, Lisa A., 1982- editor.
Title: Laryngeal cancer : an interdisciplinary resource for practitioners /
   editors, Jennifer Campion Friberg and Lisa A. Vinney.
Other titles: Laryngeal cancer (Friberg)
Description: Th orofare, NJ : SLACK Incorporated, [2017] | Includes
   bibliographical references and index.
Identifiers: LCCN 2016027004 (print) | ISBN
   9781630911591 (pbk. : alk. paper) | ISBN
Subjects: | MESH: Laryngeal Neoplasms
Classification: LCC RC280.T5 (print) | NLM WV 520 |
   DDC 616.99/422--dc23
LC record available at https://lccn.loc.gov/2016027004

ISBN: 9781630911591   (pbk)
ISBN: 9781003524762   (ebk)

DOI: 10.1201/9781003524762

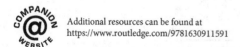

Additional resources can be found at
https://www.routledge.com/9781630911591

Dedication

To Donna Rose Campion, the inspiration for this book. While her fight with laryngeal cancer was short, her courage and grace throughout were consistently larger than life. May we learn from her, and from patients like her, that while laryngeal cancer can impact so many aspects of life, it cannot steal the ability to laugh, love, and hope.

Contents

Laryngeal Cancer: An Interdisciplinary Resource for Practitioners, includes ancillary materials specifically available for faculty use. Included are PowerPoint Slides. Please visit http://www.routledge.com/9781630911591 to obtain access.

Acknowledgments

Together, we acknowledge the support, assistance, and collaborative relationships with the many people who helped make the completion of this project a reality. Specifically, we thank the following people:

- The personnel at SLACK Incorporated for their ideas, answers, and assistance. We are particularly grateful for Brien Cummings' advice and encouragement, both of which were provided on a regular basis.
- The individual contributors for the content of this book. Individually and collectively, you endeavored to make laryngeal cancer a topic that is accessible across disciplinary and experiential boundaries. We have no doubt that your work will have tremendous impact, and we are sincerely appreciative of your efforts.
- The students who reinforced and cheered our interest in co-editing a resource focused on laryngeal cancer. Specifically, we extend gratitude to Savannah Little for her careful observations and detail-oriented work, which undoubtedly improved the quality of this book.

Dr. Friberg acknowledges the following people, who inspired this book:

- Drs. Karen Pitman and Rebecca Armendariz, physicians at Banner M.D. Anderson Cancer Center in Gilbert, Arizona. Your compassion, approachability, wisdom, and professionalism were truly bright spots at an otherwise difficult time. My family is truly appreciative for all you have done and all you continue to do.
- Shelley Campion Secrest. Whether near or far, your advice and willingness to listen are always very appreciated, as are our continued shenanigans.
- Michael, Andrew, and Molly Friberg. The words "thank you" are grossly insufficient to acknowledge the patience and support you have provided over the last several years. The three of you have sterling character and hearts of true gold. This book has been a labor of love for all of us in so many ways.
- Robert Campion. Your grit, determination, and wholesale dedication to Mom and to our family have been a true bright light that has shone particularly brightly the last 2 years. If love alone could cure laryngeal cancer, Mom would have been healthy moments after her diagnosis, thanks to you.

Dr. Vinney acknowledges the following people:

- Chad Millar. Your patience, love, and companionship over the last several years have meant more to me than you can ever know.
- Les, Linda, and Cynthia Vinney. Thank you for being my strongest and most enthusiastic supporters and for inspiring me now and throughout my life.
- Julia Foster. You have given me perspective, encouragement, and some really great laughs when I needed them most.

About the Editors

Jennifer Campion Friberg, EdD, CCC-SLP/L, ASHA Fellow is the Cross Endowed Chair in the Scholarship of Teaching and Learning and is an Associate Professor of Communication Sciences and Disorders at Illinois State University in Normal, Illinois. She has been a practicing speech-language pathologist for 18 years, working predominantly with preschool- and school-aged children with language impairments. Her teaching and research interests include language assessment, interprofessional practice in laryngeal cancer care, and the scholarship of teaching and learning.

Lisa A. Vinney, PhD, CCC-SLP/L is an Assistant Professor of Communication Sciences and Disorders at Illinois State University in Normal, Illinois. Her teaching interests include assessment and treatment of the normal and disordered voice, vocal health education and preventive care, medical speech-language pathology, and counseling. Her research focuses on the role of self-regulatory capacity, personality, and task variables on vocal behavior modification, the influence of voice on impressions, and the scholarship of teaching and learning.

Contributing Authors

Julia R. Brennan, BSE (Chapter 8)
University of Michigan Medical School
Ann Arbor, Michigan

Lisa Crujido, MS, CCC-SLP (Chapter 4)
Mayo Clinic
Department of Otorhinolaryngology
Phoenix, Arizona

Philip C. Doyle, PhD, CCC-SLP (Chapter 5)
Western University
Department of Otolaryngology–Head & Neck
    Surgery
School of Communication Sciences and
    Disorders
London, Ontario, Canada

Katharine E. Duckworth, PhD (Chapter 7)
Wake Forest Baptist Medical Center
Department Medice, Section of Hematology
    and Oncology
Comprehensive Cancer Center of Wake Forest
    University
Winston-Salem, North Carolina

Amy E. Engelhoven, PhD, CCC-SLP
    (Chapter 2)
Baldwin Wallace University
Department of Communication Sciences and
    Disorders
Berea, Ohio

Tessa Goldsmith, MA, CCC-SLP
    (Chapter 6)
Massachusetts General Hospital
Department of Speech, Language and
    Swallowing Disorders
Boston, Massachusetts

Connor W. Hoban, BS (Chapter 3)
University of Michigan Medical School
Ann Arbor, Michigan

Rachael E. Kammer, MS, CCC-SLP, BCS-S
    (Chapter 6)
Massachusetts General Hospital
Department of Speech, Language and
    Swallowing Disorders
Boston, Massachusetts

Richard P. McQuellon, PhD (Chapter 7)
Wake Forest Baptist Medical Center
Department of Hematology and Oncology
Comprehensive Cancer Center of Wake Forest
    University
Winston-Salem, North Carolina

Andrew J. Rosko, MD (Chapter 8)
University of Michigan Medical School
Department of Otolaryngology–Head and Neck
    Surgery
Ann Arbor, Michigan

Andrew G. Shuman, MD (Chapter 3,
    Chapter 8)
Division of Head and Neck Oncology
Department of Otolaryngology–Head and Neck
    Surgery
Co-Director, Program in Clinical Ethics
Center for Bioethics and Social Sciences in
    Medicine (CBSSM)
University of Michigan Medical School
Ann Arbor, Michigan

Bonnie K. Slavych, MS, CCC-SLP
    (Chapter 2)
University of Arkansas for Medical Sciences
Department of Speech-Language Pathology
Little Rock, Arkansas

Paul L. Swiecicki, MD (Chapter 3)
University of Michigan Health System
Division of Hematology and Oncology
Department of Internal Medicine
Ann Arbor, Michigan

Foreword

Cancer. This single word changes the life of a patient and his or her family, friends, and colleagues forever. No other word sends shock waves through the body in the same fashion. No other word brings with it the uncertainty of life lost, the lifelong fear of recurrence even after having been cured for many years, and the unforeseen changes as a result of the life-saving treatments administered. Once the word has been uttered, patients and families experience a whirlwind of decisions about where to receive treatment; who should administer and oversee the treatment; and how to handle work, insurance, and finances, among many more day-to-day decisions.

I am honored to write this foreword. Jen and Lisa told me that although the textbook was about caring for the communication, swallowing, nutritional, and emotional needs of people who have already been diagnosed with laryngeal cancer, they did not want to ignore the role of education about and prevention of this disease. They asked me to discuss my work in early detection and education regarding the signs, symptoms, and risks for head and neck cancer, specifically, my efforts to educate primary point-of-service health care professionals on how to identify concerning signs and seek appropriate and timely referral to the proper professionals for diagnosis.

The U.S. Preventive Services Task Force has determined that there is a lack of evidence to support national screenings for head and neck cancer. In response, my team has developed a free community-based head and neck cancer screening that has directly affected the lives of more than 5,000 people who otherwise may never have been screened or educated about head and neck cancer (www.mouthandthroatcancer.org). Multiple professionals, including otolaryngologists, oral maxillofacial surgeons, radiation oncologists, and dentists, along with dental hygienists, speech-language pathologists, and medical students, provide a comprehensive multidisciplinary head and neck examination and identify risk factors of disease, such as voice or swallowing changes. They educate people about risk behavior such as tobacco use (including the use of smokeless and chewing tobacco) and alcohol use. They also educate people about a silent risk factor, human papilloma virus, which has increased the incidence of oropharyngeal cancer more than 250% since 1995.

Do our screenings make a difference? Our studies demonstrated that education reduced smoking rates by 14% in our screening participants 6 months after screening. Our studies showed that patients are not the only stakeholders in need of these educational programs. We have worked with medical students and internal medicine interns to increase their knowledge of risks and signs of head and neck cancer, with specific attention paid to improving head and neck examinations to help identify early-stage head and neck cancer, the stage at which treatment is most effective. In addition, we have worked with speech-language pathologists to increase their comfort with identifying concerning signs of head and neck cancer and talking to their patients about at-risk behavior. Decreasing the incidence and impact of this devastating disease remains our focus.

I applaud Jen and Lisa for developing this book and hope that it will become a resource for multiple professionals. Their text demonstrates a commitment to the multidisciplinary care team in the treatment of head and neck cancer, specifically cancer of the larynx. Multiple studies have found that allied health professionals who work collaboratively produce better treatment outcomes than do professionals who work independently in their separate silos of practice/specialization, where communication and collaboration are difficult. Although not a new concept, tumor boards staffed by multiple professionals whose goal it is to develop a collaborative treatment plan and to monitor progress together have been a staple in academic medical centers and those associated with the National Cancer Institute for many years. It is unfortunate that this is not the case in all medical settings. Perhaps this book can be the impetus for teams to develop multidisciplinary care plans managed by all interested parties in fluid-communication environments providing the best care for people with laryngeal cancer.

Edie R. Hapner, PhD, CCC-SLP
Board Member, A Voice for Hope: United in the Battle Against Head and Neck Cancer
Marietta, Georgia
Full Professor, University of Southern California
Tina and Rick Caruso Department of Otolaryngology
USC Voice Center
Los Angeles, California

Introduction

It is well established that laryngeal cancer is, at best, tremendously complex, and many anatomical and physiological structures are impacted by tumors and subsequent surgical and nonsurgical treatments. Patients with laryngeal cancer often experience compromised nutrition and feeding, oral communication, and respiratory functions. The complex consequences of this disease necessitate the collaboration of professionals from multiple medical specialties (e.g., physicians, surgeons, speech-language pathologists, respiratory therapists) to provide patients with high-quality evidence-based treatment.

This book emerged from my mother's diagnosis of advanced-stage laryngeal cancer not long ago. As a speech-language pathologist, I had some knowledge of laryngeal cancer, but it became rapidly evident that I would need to learn a great deal more. In helping coordinate my mother's care, I sought a comprehensive resource for my family to better understand the multifaceted nature of laryngeal cancer; however, there seemed to be few options that were adequate in scope or detail for our needs. Thus, I reached out to colleagues in speech-language pathology, respected experts in the field of laryngeal cancer treatment, for assistance and support. No one was aware of the type of resource my family sought, and none knew of a book with supplemental resources specifically designed for patients and families to better understand laryngeal cancer management. Discussions with them led to the conception of this book.

This book is intended to serve as a valuable interprofessional resource for professionals involved in the care of people with laryngeal cancer and their families, providing readers with a comprehensive view of laryngeal cancer across specialists and specialties. It is our sincere hope that the content of this book will highlight the nuanced roles and responsibilities of professionals in the management of laryngeal cancer. These duties, specific to various disciplines, are presented as being unique but complementary, enabling the benefits of team-based laryngeal cancer management to be made clearly evident.

This book is organized in a manner consistent with the experiences of a typical patient with laryngeal cancer, moving from diagnosis through treatment to pain management. An introduction to members of the cancer care team (Chapter 1) and to the anatomy and physiology of the larynx (Chapter 2) provide a foundation for the remainder of this book, wherein topics critical to understanding laryngeal cancer are discussed: the medical and surgical diagnosis of laryngeal cancer (Chapter 3), airway/respiratory (Chapter 4), communication (Chapter 5), and nutritional/swallowing (Chapter 6) challenges for patients with laryngeal cancer, and information about counseling (Chapter 7) and palliative care (Chapter 8). Although each of these chapters can stand alone as important resources, it is through the integration of these topics that laryngeal cancer can be understood best. Italics are used throughout this text to designate terms that are defined in the glossary. Instructor materials have been created to accompany each chapter in this book. These materials summarize the most important points in each chapter and provide an outline for considering laryngeal cancer across the continuum of care.

Throughout this book, the chapter authors highlight the notion that patients and their families are critically important members of the laryngeal cancer care team. To that end, when discussing the structure and content of this book, we found it necessary to consider the unique educational needs of patients with laryngeal cancer and their families as a purposeful part of our project design. We wanted to ensure that patients and their families had access to information about laryngeal cancer management that was straightforward, informative, and valuable. Thus, a collection of supplemental materials was created to summarize and extend chapter information to form brief non-technical references to explain complicated medical information. These supplemental resources have been designed to support an important mission, which was to gather useful information to help answer important questions and facilitate conversations between all stakeholders to positively affect the quality of life for patients with laryngeal cancer and their families.

Please visit the companion website for this text at (www.routledge.com/9781630911591/books/laryngealcancerforms). This companion website includes supplemental materials that are intended for use by patients and families of patients with laryngeal cancer. Specifically, this companion website includes resources which correspond to chapters in this text and includes:

- Brief chapter summaries as an overview of important information
- Useful references, figures, and tables concerning the interdisciplinary care of patients with laryngeal cancer
- Guidance in asking specific questions for allied health personnel

I truly believe that the combination of this book and its supplemental materials provides a rich and comprehensive resource for the support of patients with laryngeal cancer. I hope you, as a reader, will agree.

Jennifer Campion Friberg, EdD, CCC-SLP/L, ASHA Fellow

1

The Laryngeal Cancer Care Team
Diagnosis Through Treatment

Lisa A. Vinney, PhD, CCC-SLP/L and
Jennifer Campion Friberg, EdD, CCC-SLP/L, ASHA Fellow

This chapter serves as a foundation for the remainder of this book and is intended to introduce the interdisciplinary team tasked with caring for patients with laryngeal cancer (LC). While subsequent chapters detail specific aspects of LC diagnosis and management (e.g., respiration, communication, swallowing, counseling, and pain management), this chapter provides a general overview of the process of diagnosing LC and explains the roles of the medical professionals who assist patients with LC from diagnosis through treatment. The trajectory of one patient, Rose, is highlighted to facilitate this discussion (Case Study 1-1).

DIAGNOSTIC PROCESS

The diagnostic process for LC begins the moment that suspicious symptoms are noted (Box 1-1) and an evaluation plan is formed to determine their impact on a patient's health and well-being. Rose's case illustrates some of the common signs and symptoms that may lead to an evaluation of the *larynx* (Box 1-2). Because of the loss of important function that is evident in the early stages of LC (e.g., eating, communicating with a strong *voice*), many cases (approximately 60%) of LC are diagnosed very early (American Cancer Society [ACS], 2015a; Hoffman et al., 2006). That said, LC that is discovered in a later vs early stage of the disease is likely to result in more severe voice, swallowing, and respiratory impairments.

A variety of individuals may be involved in the diagnosis of LC, although it is important to acknowledge that differences exist in the path that patients take to an eventual LC diagnosis. Some patients may notice symptoms on their own that lead them to seek medical help (i.e., hoarseness, *dysphagia, dyspnea*), whereas others may have suspicious growths identified during routine medical or dental visits or as part of testing and treatments for other conditions. Thus, all or only some of the professionals described here may be involved in the diagnosis of LC, depending on each patient's circumstances.

Friberg, J. C., & Vinney, L. A.
Laryngeal Cancer: An Interdisciplinary
Resource for Practitioners (pp. 1-13).
© 2017 Taylor and Francis Group.

CASE STUDY 1-1

PATIENT NAME: ROSE

Clinical Status: referred for magnetic resonance imaging (MRI)

    Rose, a 64-year-old long-term smoker, experienced a gradual onset of suspicious symptoms over the course of several months. Initially, she began to notice that her voice was raspy and hoarse. She and her *primary care physician* (PCP) attributed this status change to continued issues with gastroesophageal reflux disease. Her medicine was changed, yet her voice did not improve in intensity or quality. Around the same time, Rose began to notice difficulty swallowing foods that had never been problematic in the past (e.g., crackers, toast, apples). In response to this difficulty, she started eating softer foods and eventually found that even those were difficult to swallow. These dysphagia symptoms led to a referral from her PCP to an ear, nose, and throat (ENT) doctor. After completing a basic examination of Rose and considering her long history of smoking and current symptom profile, the ENT was interested in determining whether a tumor in her larynx may have been compromising her ability to eat and communicate effectively. The ENT immediately referred Rose for MRI to establish the presence or absence or LC.

BOX 1-1

COMMON RISK FACTORS FOR LARYNGEAL CANCER

- History of smoking
- History of alcohol use
- Poor nutrition
- Human papillomavirus infection
- Exposure to noxious chemicals or irritants in the workplace
- Genetic syndromes (Fanconi anemia or dyskeratosis 18)
- Sex (more common in males than in females)
- Age (most common in patients older than 65 years)

American Cancer Society, 2015D

Primary Care Physicians

    PCPs play an important role in the initial assessment and diagnosis of LC because patients often approach their PCP with their initial LC symptoms. In fact, Alho, Teppo, Mäntyselkä, and Kantola (2006) estimate that 11% of patients seen annually by their PCP present with symptoms consistent with a diagnosis of LC, although only a small fraction of these patients are ever diagnosed with LC, as LC symptoms can be indicative of other, less serious illnesses. Thus, it is important for PCPs to combine their knowledge of a patient's social, behavioral, and medical history with their clinical presentation to make appropriate referrals to specialists and maximize opportunities for an accurate and timely diagnosis of LC (Alho et al., 2006).

BOX 1-2

COMMON SYMPTOMS OF LARYNGEAL CANCER

- Persistent sore throat
- Hoarse voice
- Chronic cough
- Pain when swallowing
- Difficulty swallowing
- Ear pain
- Difficulty breathing
- Weight loss
- Lump or mass in the neck region

American Cancer Society, 2015E

Otolaryngologists

Otolaryngologists are often called ENTs because they provide medical and surgical interventions for diseases of the ears, nose, and throat. Patients with LC may be referred to an ENT who has completed specialty fellowship training in surgical head and neck *oncology* (i.e., surgical interventions for cancer of the head and neck) and laryngology (i.e., diagnosis and management of the larynx; American Academy of Otolaryngology–Head and Neck Surgery, 2014). As was the case with Rose (see Case Study 1-1), a patient who displays signs and symptoms of LC is often referred by his or her PCP to an ENT. In particular, after a full ear, nose, and throat physical examination (i.e., neck palpation, observation of the oropharyngeal cavity with the use of a tongue depressor, etc.), video imaging or rigid oral/flexible nasal endoscopy of the larynx, using a strong light source and magnification, will take place. Then, the ENT may collect tissue samples from the larynx and pharynx for *biopsy* if a suspicious growth(s) is visualized during imaging or felt during the physical examination. In conjunction with other physicians and the results of additional testing, the ENT is likely to make the initial LC diagnosis, stage the severity, make treatment recommendations, and discuss treatment options with the patient and his or her family on the basis of the severity of the LC diagnosis.

After a diagnosis of LC, an ENT with fellowship training in surgical head and neck oncology might perform procedures to excise laryngeal tumors, remove part or all of the larynx, and/or complete reconstructive surgery. These physicians also monitor the laryngeal site during and after treatments for LC because complications from tumor location and nonsurgical and/or surgical treatments for tumors may compromise phonation, swallowing, or breathing. These complications may necessitate additional medical intervention from an ENT. Overall, ENTs play a central role in the diagnosis, treatment, and follow-up of patients with LC (see Chapter 3 for more details about the role of ENTs in the diagnosis and surgical and medical management of patients with LC).

Diagnostic Radiologists

A *diagnostic radiologist* is a doctor with specialized training in using imaging techniques as part of the assessment process for many diseases within the body. Specific to LC, diagnostic radiologists select and conduct tests such as MRI or *computed tomography* (CT) scans to diagnose the presence of a primary tumor in the larynx or *metastasis* to other areas of the body. A patient who shows signs and symptoms of LC may encounter a diagnostic radiologist after receiving a referral for an MRI or CT scan from his or her PCP, ENT, or other physician specialist. The imaging techniques implemented by a diagnostic radiologist allow for structures in or around the larynx that were unable to be visualized during the original head and neck examination and via endoscopy to be viewed in great detail (Blitz & Aygun, 2008). Thus, diagnostic radiologists play a key role on a multidisciplinary LC team, most notably because their findings have a strong impact on the subsequent selection and prioritization of treatment options for patients with LC by other medical professionals.

It should be noted that diagnostic radiologists do not engage in the treatment or management of LC. Rather, they are directly involved in efforts to determine the effectiveness of LC treatments through periodic monitoring via imaging (Connor, 2007).

Pathologists

Pathologists are doctors with specialized training in studying cells or tissues to provide a definitive diagnosis for conditions such as cancer. They study samples from biopsies and other clinical tests to identify cellular markers for tumors to help them diagnose and stage cancers for treatment and decision making. In the case of LC, pathologists read and interpret information from samples taken from tissue biopsies of the larynx. From their examination of the microscopic composition of cells within the laryngeal tissue, pathologists are able to determine whether cancer cells or cancer are present (Wenig, 2002). If cancerous or precancerous cells are found, they are classified by characteristics that will facilitate appropriate diagnosis and treatment. As was the case with diagnostic radiologists, pathologists are not involved directly in the treatment or management of LC in patients, but they may be involved at various stages of LC management, particularly if biopsies of other parts of the body are needed to confirm or rule out metastasis.

STAGING OF LARYNGEAL CANCERS

The physicians working with patients and their families during the diagnostic process first determine whether tumors of the larynx are *malignant* or *benign*. Then, these professionals help to assign a stage for each patient's LC to enable the patient and the LC care team to make informed decisions about treatment and disease management. The *staging of LC* can also help patients understand their long-term prognosis.

TNM TUMOR STAGING SYSTEM FOR LARYNGEAL CANCER

The staging of LC is quite detailed and depends completely on whether the LC tumor is considered to be *supraglottic* (superior to the *vocal folds*), *glottic* (at the level of the vocal folds/glottis), or *subglottic* (inferior to the level of the vocal folds). The location of an LC tumor is a critical consideration for staging because the impact of a tumor in one location will affect the physiology and functions of the head and neck differently than a tumor in another location. Because many of the staging criteria are based entirely on these effects on physiology and function, specificity is crucial for assigning an accurate stage for any LC.

To manage this complex process, the ACS (2015b) advocates use of the TNM system, which was developed by the American Joint Committee on Cancer (Figure 1-1). Physicians can assign an LC stage on the basis of a combination of factors, including tumor location and size (T), *lymph node involvement* (N), and metastasis (M), by using the following system:

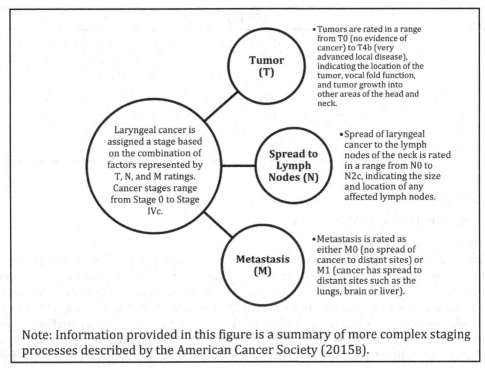

Note: Information provided in this figure is a summary of more complex staging processes described by the American Cancer Society (2015b).

Figure 1-1. Staging for LC.

- Tumors are rated in a range from stage T0 (no tumor can be found) to stage T4b (tumor is growing into the spinal area, surrounds the carotid artery, or has grown into the area between the patient's lungs). Each patient's T rating indicates the degree to which vocal fold function is compromised, the location of the primary LC tumor, and its growth into other areas of the head and neck. By indicating the size, spread, and location of the tumor, the T rating also provides information about the tumor's effect on important functions such as breathing and swallowing.

- Any spread of LC to the lymph nodes of the neck (N) is rated in a range from N0 (no evidence of cancer spread to lymph nodes) to N3 (cancer has spread to at least one lymph node that is larger than 6 cm across). The N rating provides information on the specific size and location of any affected lymph nodes.

- Metastasis (M) is rated as one of two values to indicate the presence (M1) or absence (M0) of cancer spread from an original LC site to an area such as the lungs, brain, or liver.

Once a patient has been assigned T, N, and M values in accordance with his or her LC imaging, symptoms, and evaluation results, this information is combined to assign an overall stage for the cancer (Box 1-3). Stages of LC range from 0 through IVC. The ACS (2015a) presents the following rules to reflect the combination of T, N, and M values for each LC stage:

- Stage 0: Tis, N0, M0

- Stage I: T1, N0, M0

- Stage II: T2, N0, M0

- Stage III: T3, N0, M0, or T1 to T3, N1, M0

BOX 1-3

The staging information for LC provided in this chapter is a summary of a very complex process. For detailed information about the differences in cancer staging for supraglottic, glottic, and subglottic LCs, please refer to the following resources:

- The American Cancer Society: http://www.cancer.org/cancer/laryngealandhypopharyngealcancer/detailedguide/laryngeal-and-hypopharyngeal-cancer-staging
- National Cancer Institute: http://www.cancer.gov/types/head-and-neck/hp/laryngeal-treatment-pdq#section/_13

- Stage IVA: T4a, N0 or N1, M0, or T1 to T4a, N2, M0
- Stage IVB: T4b, any N, M0, or any T, N3, M0
- Stage IVC: any T, any N, M1

In general, earlier-stage cancers result in better overall outcomes in terms of retaining function of the laryngeal physiology and for patient survival (Lester & Yang, 2012). This is especially true, given that LC caught in its early stages will typically require less invasive and/or toxic treatments, which results in fewer compromises to overall health (Plenderleith, 1990). Later-stage LC is associated with more complex treatments and greater declines in functions such as swallowing and phonation. Patients with later-stage LC typically require involvement from a greater number of medical and allied health practitioners to maximize the benefits and minimize the adverse effects of medical or surgical treatments (Case Study 1-2).

AFTER LARYNGEAL CANCER DIAGNOSIS

The presentation of LC can negatively affect the life-sustaining functions of airway protection, swallowing, feeding, and breathing. This condition also affects oral communication, a function closely connected with quality of life and interpersonal relationships. Unfortunately, because the larynx is vital to all of these major functions, treatment decisions that affect function in this region are incredibly complex (Forastiere, Weber, & Trotti, 2015; Tomeh & Holsinger, 2014; Tufano & Stafford, 2008). As is illustrated in Rose's case (see Case Study 1-1), the consequences of this disease necessitate the collaboration of multiple medical specialists (e.g., physicians representing various medical specialties, *speech-language pathologists* [SLPs], *respiratory therapists* [RTs]) to provide patients with high-quality evidence-based treatment. Indeed, the multidisciplinary team approach to serving patients with LC is considered best practice (Bhatti & Tufano, 2008; Forastiere et al., 2003; Lester & Yang, 2012).

After diagnosis, the primary consideration of a patient with LC and the LC care team is whether to pursue one of two main treatment options: surgical intervention involving *partial* or *total laryngectomy* or targeted medical management including *chemotherapy* and/or *radiation*. The typical primary focus after LC diagnosis is to eradicate as much of the tumor as possible using a medical or surgical approach despite the impact of such treatment on communication, swallowing, and breathing. With this fact in mind, the initial meetings between patients with LC, their families, and the treatment team generally focus on options to remove or shrink the laryngeal tumor. Such treatment options are typically presented by a team of physicians representing various areas of expertise in LC treatment. In addition to the ENT who can surgically remove the tumor(s), typically via a partial or total laryngectomy, these physicians are tasked with explaining

---

CASE STUDY 1-2

PATIENT NAME: ROSE

Clinical Status: post-MRI, making treatment decisions

After MRI was completed, Rose was diagnosed with a late-stage tumor of the larynx. She met with the ENT to discuss the results of her MRI. The ENT indicated that a total laryngectomy would be the most beneficial surgical approach to treat Rose's cancer. Beyond this recommendation, he provided the names of a radiologist and a medical oncologist with whom Rose could discuss radiation and chemotherapy as additional treatment options. This ENT was not part of a larger team of professionals who specialized in treating LC and, thus, could not provide Rose with the opportunity for collaborative consultation or to receive input from a wide variety of LC specialists as part of her decision-making process.

Rose and her family were uncomfortable with the segmentation they sensed between service providers under this ENT's model of care. Rose's daughter, a speech-language pathologist, was particularly concerned that no mention of communication, feeding, or general well-being were part of the overall discussion of Rose's disease management. As a result of these concerns, Rose pursued a second opinion with a large team-based cancer treatment center near her home.

During her first consultation with this new team, Rose and her family met with an ENT, a medical oncologist, and a radiation oncologist. Together, these professionals presented the advantages and disadvantages of each possible treatment approach. Rose's family was included in this consultation, as was a *social worker* to assist Rose in managing her medical care, a speech-language pathologist to address concerns about feeding and communication, and a *palliative care physician* to begin conversations about pain management and living a functional life with LC.

The differences between a team-based and a non–team-based approach to LC care were evident to Rose and her family, and ultimately, they chose to pursue treatment with a dedicated team of medical specialists rather than to put their own care team together through the use of unaffiliated specialists. For Rose and her family, it was important to have her medical care team operate as a unit, to observe these individuals in consultation with each other regularly, and to enjoy the feeling of a cohesive approach to her care.

---

the diagnosis, staging assignment, and treatment options for patients with LC. These physicians represent a variety of specialties, as described later.

Radiation Oncologists

A *radiation oncologist* is a doctor with specialized training in the treatment of cancer via radiation. A radiation oncologist identifies the type and dosage of radiation appropriate for each patient with LC. Often, radiation oncologists collaborate with *medical oncologists* to treat patients with *chemoradiation*, a combination of radiation and chemotherapy.

Radiation can be used to treat LC in any of the following ways (ACS, 2015c):

- As the main treatment for LC
- As a preliminary treatment for patients who are not good candidates for immediate surgery

- As a treatment after surgery to attack any remaining cancer cells after a partial/total laryngectomy

- As a palliative treatment to reduce the severity of symptoms in patients with advanced LC

Because patients who receive radiation therapies for LC often suffer from treatment effects such as dermatologic problems, dry mouth, swelling, difficulty swallowing, respiratory concerns, and fatigue, radiation oncologists often work with other allied medical professionals to mitigate these symptoms so that patients can tolerate full courses of radiation treatment as comfortably as possible (ACS, 2015c) (see Chapter 3 for additional information on the role of the radiation oncologist in the management of LC).

Medical Oncologists

A medical oncologist is a doctor with specialized training in treating cancers through the use of pharmacological agents such as chemotherapy (Case Study 1-3). Medical oncologists will recommend dosages and frequencies of these pharmacological agents for LC care depending on the stage of the disease and other treatments received by the patient (see Chapter 3 for additional information on the role of the medical oncologist in the management of LC).

Allied Health Professionals

As exemplified with Rose's case, once a patient has worked with medical doctors to select the best treatment for the LC, he or she often requires support from other allied health professionals to ensure that needs relative to ongoing medical issues, communication, nutrition, and pain management are addressed adequately. These allied health professionals complete the LC management team and are routinely involved in helping patients manage the effects of the cancer and secondary effects from medical and surgical management.

Speech-Language Pathologists

An SLP is a professional who receives specialized training in the assessment and management of *speech*, language, and swallowing problems (American Speech-Language-Hearing Association, 2007). Often, SLPs work with patients with LC to minimize functional alterations in communication, breathing, and eating. They can help patients communicate through their own voice or through the use of other techniques after surgery, with feeding-modality decisions, and with airway issues (Starmer, Tippett, & Webster, 2008). Referral to an SLP is appropriate when the management of LC compromises a patient's ability to communicate effectively or swallow safely (see Chapters 4, 5, and 6 for additional information on the role of the SLP in managing respiration, communication, and swallowing in patients with LC).

Gastroenterologists

A *gastroenterologist* focuses on diseases and dysfunction that affect the gastrointestinal (GI) tract, which contains organs for transporting and consuming food material, absorbing nutrients, and ridding the body of waste. Patients with LC commonly have dysfunction in the transit of food through their GI system because of swallowing dysfunction (dysphagia), which requires surgical or medical interventions from a GI physician. Gastroenterologists may prescribe medication, dilate the *esophagus* to widen it and enable better food transit into the stomach, or perform surgery to remove obstructions in the GI tract. These doctors may also place feeding tubes in patients who cannot swallow food safely to ensure that they receive adequate nutrition during and/or after treatment (see Chapter 6 for some additional information on these interventions in the context of swallowing and nutritional challenges faced by patients with LC).

CASE STUDY 1-3

PATIENT NAME: ROSE

Clinical Status: undergoing first round of chemoradiation

After extensive consultation with her LC team, Rose and her family understood that surgery was not the best option for her on the basis of the size and location of her tumor. Rather, a medical approach combining chemotherapy and radiation were thought to be the most effective first stage of her LC treatment.

Shortly after radiation and chemotherapy started, a combination of tumor growth and swelling from her treatments necessitated Rose to undergo a tracheotomy to restore her full respiratory capabilities and to have a gastric feeding tube placed to maintain a consistent and safe method of feeding. At that point in her treatment, Rose began to take advantage of the specialists on her LC team to keep her comfortable and moving toward the quality of life she was seeking. An RT was integral in training her and her family on tracheostomy care. A speech-language pathologist assisted in assessing Rose for alternative methods of oral communication. A *dietitian* monitored her caloric intake. A physician assistant checked on her daily to ensure that all aspects of her care were well coordinated. As Rose recovered from her tracheotomy and feeding tube placement and planned to return home, a social worker helped to coordinate home care and arrange for a consult with a palliative care doctor to assist her in coping with the adverse effects of her treatments and surgeries.

Eventually, as her tumor continued to grow, it became evident that Rose's LC was aggressive and resistant to her ongoing curative treatments. An MRI scan shortly after Rose's tracheotomy indicated metastasis of the LC to both lungs. With the support of her family, Rose made the very difficult decision to discontinue all attempts at curative treatment for her LC. At this point, her palliative care doctor and social worker became central to her care, collaborating to arrange for hospice support, home health care, and pain management. The support of these professionals enabled Rose and her family to focus on spending time together rather than worrying about her end-of-life care.

Oncology Nurses/Nurse Practitioners

An *oncology nurse* has specialized training and experience in caring for patients with cancer and specifically administering chemotherapy to patients. Oncology nurses practice alongside surgical, radiation, and medical oncologists and are instrumental in patient assessment, patient education, management of patient symptoms, supportive patient/family care, direct patient care, and coordination of care (Rieger & Yarbro, 2003).

Respiratory Therapists

RTs are allied health professionals who treat people suffering from breathing problems. Patients with LC who undergo surgical removal of all or part of their larynx or with tumor invasion into the *trachea* will experience changes in the structure and function of their respiratory system. RTs provide support for airway management in a number of ways. For example, they may provide artificial ventilation or suction the airway to clear it of secretions and maintain its patency. They are also particularly involved in advising patients on proper care and maintenance of their airway after *tracheotomy* (see Chapter 4 for additional information on the role of RTs in airway management).

Dietitians

Dietitians are allied health professionals who assess patients' nutritional requirements and whether they are being met. They treat nutritional deficiencies by creating and adjusting nutrition treatment plans. Dietitians may also determine the particular method and contents of tube feeds or intravenous fluids if they are required. Patients with LC often have difficulty chewing and swallowing food or doing so safely (because of the risk of *aspiration*) due to the location of tumors in their larynx or hardening of tissue around their neck after radiation. In either of these situations, dietitians may work closely with an SLP to coordinate safe and adequate nutritional intake (see Chapter 6 for additional information on the role of dietitians in nutritional management in patients with LC).

Clinical Psychologists, Social Workers, Counselors, and Therapists

Clinical psychologists, social workers, and counselors/therapists are licensed professionals who provide comprehensive mental health care services (American Counseling Association, 2015; American Psychological Association, 2015; National Association of Social Workers, 2015). Clinical psychologists are doctoral-level professionals who provide individual and group health counseling to support mental health needs and can diagnose psychological disorders (e.g., depression, anxiety) specifically through the administration and scoring of a wide range of psychological tests. Their training often has a strong focus on research and the scientific method in addition to psychological theory.

Licensed clinical social workers (LCSWs), licensed practical counselors (LPCs), licensed mental health counselors (LMCHs), and marriage and family therapists (MFTs) are masters-level professionals who diagnose and treat mental health conditions through a more limited range of assessment approaches than do psychologists and through counseling, respectively. Unlike some of the other professionals described here, social workers may focus on providing case management and advocacy services instead of counseling, depending on their role on the multidisciplinary cancer care team and their training and specialization. Regardless of their title, education, and training, all of the professionals discussed here typically engage in talking and listening to patients with LC to empower them to improve their well-being and mental health (Kaplan, Tarvydas, & Gladding, 2013) (see Chapter 7 for additional information on counseling patients with LC).

Psychiatrists/Psychiatric-Mental Health Nurse Practitioner

Psychiatrists are physicians who diagnose and treat psychological conditions by prescribing medications to improve psychological functioning while monitoring side effects, dosage, and interactions with other prescriptions (American Psychiatric Association, 2016; Arehart-Treichel, 2012). *Psychiatric-mental health nurse* practitioners are registered nurses with postgraduate training in mental health conditions who may prescribe medication and other medical interventions for psychological conditions (American Psychiatric Nurses Association, 2015). Psychiatrists and mental health nurse practitioners may also provide counseling or talk therapy, but their training and experience are typically focused on the medical and pharmacological management of psychiatric conditions.

In contrast to psychologists, therapists, social workers, and counselors, neither psychiatrists nor psychiatric-mental health nurse practitioners typically perform paper-and-pencil psychological testing. In terms of client management, counselors, therapists, and social workers may focus on counseling, whereas psychiatrists and psychiatric nurse practitioners may focus on medical management. It is also possible for psychiatrists or psychiatric nurse practitioners to perform both counseling and medical management for psychological concerns in patients with cancer. Although the roles of these professionals may overlap sometimes, one of the most important considerations for patients with LC who seek mental health services is ascertaining whether these practitioners have specialized knowledge in psychosocial oncology. Psychosocial oncology (American Psychosocial Oncology Society, 2015) is a subspecialty of oncology that focuses on the impact of cancer on the psychosocial functioning of patients and their families throughout the disease process.

PAIN MANAGEMENT, QUALITY OF LIFE, AND PALLIATIVE CARE

As was the case with Rose, most patients with LC will likely experience the need for some sort of pain management at some point in their disease process. Thus, the final member of the LC care team is a palliative care physician. A palliative care physician has specialized training in the management of physical and emotional pain or debilitating symptoms of chronic or serious illnesses such as cancer (American Academy of Hospice and Palliative Medicine, 2015). Although palliative care doctors are associated most closely with end-of-life care, they can be valuable members of the LC team at any point during LC management. To this end, these specialists provide support for both curative (nonhospice) and end-of-life (hospice) care for patients with a variety of diseases, including LC.

The main role of a palliative care specialist is ultimately to ensure that each patient with LC is able to maintain the quality of life he or she desires, for as long as possible. Palliative care specialists work with patients and their families to determine individualized priorities for care and indicators of quality of life. In Rose's case, the palliative care physician played an increasingly central role on her LC care team because the metastasis of LC to her lungs meant that Rose's cancer was no longer curable. As such, discussions with her treatment team led to the decision to discontinue chemoradiation treatments and initiate palliative hospice-based care for her. Rose and her family were able to work closely with her palliative care doctor to ensure that her needs and desires were prioritized in her end-of-life care (see Chapter 8 for more information on the role of the palliative care physician in LC care).

CONCLUSION

Ideally, the medical specialists who work with patients with LC practice as a dynamic, multidisciplinary team that is able to individualize care and address patient and family priorities across all aspects of diagnosis and treatment for LC. The different skills of each professional are complementary in nature. Thus, because of the complexity of the LC diagnosis and treatment, no single professional can or should be tasked with its complete diagnosis and management. In addition, because the needs of patients are paramount to LC treatment, an individualized multidisciplinary approach to patient care is both desirable and necessary for best addressing disease presentation, quality-of-life priorities, and overall prognosis. Ultimately, when a team approach is implemented, the best chance for proper diagnosis and life-sustaining treatments can be encouraged by doctors and other medical specialists coordinating care to work toward successful treatment for patients with LC. However, a team approach is equally important for cases in which a cure for LC is not possible because the palliation of suffering can be prioritized and an emphasis on patient-determined quality of life can be honored in a coordinated effort to address specific patient desires. Thus, it is through the active collaboration of all the professionals described in this chapter—across all LC types, stages, and treatments—that best practice in the diagnosis and treatment of LC can be realized.

REFERENCES

Alho, O., Teppo, H., Mäntyselkä, P., & Kantola, S. (2006). Head and neck cancer in primary care: Presenting symptoms and the effect of delayed diagnosis of cancer cases. *Canadian Medical Association Journal, 174*, 779–784.

American Academy of Hospice and Palliative Medicine. (2015). AAHPM and the specialty of hospice and palliative medicine. Retrieved from http://aahpm.org/about/about.

American Academy of Otolaryngology–Head and Neck Surgery. (2014). About us. Retrieved from http://www.entnet.org/content/about-us.

American Cancer Society. (2015a). Can laryngeal and hypopharyngeal cancers be found early? Retrieved from http://www.cancer.org/cancer/laryngealandhypopharyngealcancer/detailedguide/laryngeal-and-hypopharyngeal-cancer-detection.

American Cancer Society. (2015b). How are laryngeal and hypopharyngeal cancers staged? Retrieved from http://www.cancer.org/cancer/laryngealandhypopharyngealcancer/detailedguide/laryngeal-and-hypopharyngeal-cancer-staging.

American Cancer Society. (2015c). Radiation therapy for laryngeal and hypopharyngeal cancers. Retrieved from http://www.cancer.org/cancer/laryngealandhypopharyngealcancer/detailedguide/laryngeal-and-hypopharyngeal-cancer-treating-radiation.

American Cancer Society. (2015d). Signs and symptoms of laryngeal and hypolaryngeal cancers. Retrieved from http://www.cancer.org/cancer/laryngealandhypopharyngealcancer/detailedguide/laryngeal-and-hypopharyngeal-cancer-signs-symptoms.

American Cancer Society. (2015e). What are the risk factors for laryngeal and hypopharyngeal cancers? Retrieved from http://www.cancer.org/cancer/laryngealandhypopharyngealcancer/detailedguide/laryngeal-and-hypo-pharyngeal-cancer-risk-factors.

American Counseling Association. (2015). Our mission. Retrieved from https://www.counseling.org/about-us/about-aca/our-mission.

American Psychiatric Association. (2016). What is Psychiatry? Retrieved from https://www.psychiatry.org/patients-families/what-is-psychiatry

American Psychiatric Nurses Association. (2015). About psychiatric-mental health nurses. Retrieved from http://www.apna.org/i4a/pages/index.cfm?pageid=3292.

American Psychological Association. (2015). Clinical psychology. Retrieved from http://www.apa.org/ed/graduate/specialize/clinical.aspx.

American Psychosocial Oncology Society. (2015). What is psychosocial oncology? Retrieved from https://www.apos-society.org/APOS/People_Affected_by_Cancer/What_is_Psychosocial.aspx.

American Speech-Language-Hearing Association. (2007). Scope of practice in speech-language pathology. Retrieved from http://www.asha.org/policy/SP2007-00283.htm.

Arehart-Treichel, J. (2012). Cancer patients have much to gain from psychiatric treatment. *Psychiatric news.* Retrieved from http://psychnews.psychiatryonline.org/doi/10.1176/pn.47.6.psychnews_47_6_14-a.

Bhatti, N., & Tufano, R. P. (2008). Preface. *Otolaryngologic Clinics of North America, 41*, xi–xii.

Blitz, A. M., & Aygun, N. (2008). Radiologic evaluation of larynx cancer. *Otolaryngologic Clinics of North America, 41*, 697–713.

Connor, S. (2007). Laryngeal cancer: How does the radiologist help? *Cancer Imaging, 7*, 93–103.

Forastiere, A. A., Goepfert, H., Maor, M., Pajak, T. F., Weber, R., Morrison, W., … Cooper, J. (2003). Concurrent chemotherapy and radiotherapy for organ preservation in advanced laryngeal cancer. *New England Journal of Medicine, 349*, 2091–2098.

Forastiere, A. A., Weber, R. S., & Trotti, A. (2015). Organ preservation for advanced larynx cancer: Issues and outcomes. *Journal of Clinical Oncology, 33*, 3262–3268.

Hoffman, H. T., Porter, K., Karnell, L., Cooper, J. S., Weber, R. S., Langer, C. J., … Robinson, R. A. (2006). Laryngeal cancer in the United States: Changes in demographics, patterns of care, and survival. *The Laryngoscope, 116*, 1–13.

Kaplan, D. M., Tarvydas, V. M., & Gladding, S. T. (2013). 20/20: A vision for the future of counseling: The new consensus definition of counseling. *Journal of Counseling and Development, 92*, 366–372

Lester, S., & Yang, W.-Y. (2012). Principles and management of head and neck cancer. *Surgery, 30*, 617–623.

National Association of Social Workers. (2015). Clinical social work. Retrieved from http://www.naswdc.org/practice/clinical/default.asp.

Plenderleith, I. H. (1990). Treating the treatment: Toxicity of cancer chemotherapy. *Canadian Family Physician, 36*, 1827–1830.

Rieger, P. T., & Yarbro, C. H. (2003). Role of the oncology nurse. In D. W. Kufe, R. E. Pollack, R. R. Weischselbaum, R. Bast, & T. S. Gansler, (Eds.). *Cancer review: Volume 6.* Hamilton, ON, Canada: BC Decker.

Starmer, H. M., Tippett, D. C., & Webster, K. T. (2008). Effects of laryngeal cancer on voice and swallowing. *Otolaryngologic Clinics of North America, 41*, 793–818.

Tomeh, C., & Holsinger, C. F. (2014). Laryngeal cancer. *Current Opinion in Otolaryngology & Head and Neck Surgery, 22,* 147–153.

Tufano, R. P., & Stafford, E. M. (2008). Organ preservation surgery for laryngeal cancer. *Otolaryngologic Clinics of North America, 41,* 741–755.

Wenig, B. M. (2002). Squamous cell carcinoma of the upper aerodigestive tract: Precursors and problematic variants. *Modern Pathology, 15,* 229–254.

Understanding the Anatomy and Physiology of Speech, Voice, and Swallowing

Amy E. Engelhoven, PhD, CCC-SLP and
Bonnie K. Slavych, MS, CCC-SLP

The oral-motor system, human larynx, and respiratory systems are central to speech, chewing and swallowing, voice, and respiration and are commonly affected by laryngeal cancer (LC). This chapter provides the reader with a broad introduction to the normal structure of these systems and their major role in the previously noted functions. Thus, this content should serve as foundation for understanding how LC and its management may compromise basic life-sustaining functions, communication, and quality of life.

ANATOMY AND PHYSIOLOGY OF THE ORAL-MOTOR SYSTEM

The oral-motor system works together with the larynx and respiratory system to enable speech, swallowing, and breathing. It is composed of articulators, which may be mobile or immobile and which work in tandem to enable automatic and coordinated movements for swallowing and communication. In this section, the anatomical organization and functions of this system, and its roles in swallowing, phonation, and speech, are discussed.

Oral, Nasal, and Pharyngeal Cavities

The oral cavity and pharynx can be classified as a tunnel system with surrounding walls that constrict and release for swallowing, resonance, sound production, and respiration. The oral cavity extends from the lips to the faucial pillars (fauces) in the back of the mouth. The ceiling of the mouth includes a hard bony plate called the hard palate, which transitions to the soft palate (velum) and, finally, the uvula. The teeth and gum ridge, known as the alveolar ridge, form

Friberg, J. C., & Vinney, L. A.
Laryngeal Cancer: An Interdisciplinary
Resource for Practitioners (pp. 15-44).
© 2017 Taylor and Francis Group.

Figure 2-1. Divisions of the pharynx in context of the upper airway. (Reprinted with permission from Blausen.com staff. "Blausen gallery 2014." Wikiversity Journal of Medicine. DOI: 10.15347/wjm/2014.010. ISSN 20018762. [Own work] [CC BY 3.0 (http://creativecommons.org/licenses/by/3.0)], via Wikimedia Commons.)

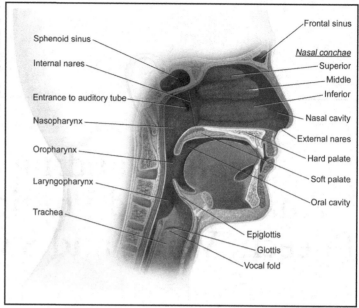

the edges of the oral cavity and contain the tooth sockets. The oral cavity is able to take on many configurations by altering the position of the lips and tongue (Zemlin, 1998). These various shapes facilitate the articulation of a great variety of speech sounds.

The buccal cavities are located on each side of the oral cavity between the back teeth and the cheeks of the face. The nasal cavity's floor is the hard palate of the oral cavity, and the pharynx is a 12-cm muscular tube that runs from the area behind the nasal cavity to the vocal folds and includes the nasopharynx, oropharynx, and hypopharynx. The nasopharynx extends from the space above the velum to the nasal turbinates toward the front of the face; the oropharyx sits below the nasopharynx and directly behind the fauces; and the laryngopharynx (or hypopharynx) has its upper border represented by the hyoid bone and its lower border represented by the opening of the esophagus. Figure 2-1 illustrates these divisions of the pharynx in the context of the oral and nasal cavities, hard and soft palates, and other related structures. Tables 2-1 through 2-5 list the muscles of the face, tongue, jaw, velum, and pharynx along with their locations and functions. Origin refers to where each muscle is fixated, and *insertion* refers to the part that moves with muscle contraction. Innervation refers to the nerve or nerve distribution that stimulates the muscle (Box 2-1).

Although the cavities within the oral-motor system facilitate the articulation of speech sounds, alterations in resonance, and manipulation of food, the muscles within this system must contract to enable these changes in shape to occur in the first place. The muscles of the lips play a particularly major role in eating and speaking. Specifically, during meals, after sensory receptors within the lips detect the food's temperature and texture, the orbicularis oris muscle then facilitates compression of the lips to draw food off of a utensil and keep it in the mouth during chewing. In addition, the risorius and buccinator muscles prevent food from pocketing between the gums and the cheeks while it is chewed and formed into a *bolus* (mass). The upper lip works quickly and contracts strongly during lip closure, whereas the lower lip is assisted in upward and downward movements by the mandible. These movements are important for chewing and swallowing and for the formation of speech sounds (see Table 2-1 for further details about major muscles of the mouth and face).

Of all of the articulators, the tongue is of utmost importance for speech and swallowing (Zemlin, 1998). The extrinsic tongue muscles are grossly responsible for tongue posture, whereas the intrinsic tongue muscles are responsible for finite movements for articulation and swallowing.

TABLE 2-1				
MUSCLES OF THE FACE AND MOUTH				
MUSCLE	**ORIGIN**	**INSERTION**	**INNERVATION**	**FUNCTION**
Orbicularis oris	Corner of lips	Opposite corner of lips	Cranial nerve VII (facial nerve)	Closes and protrudes lips
Risorius	Posterior area of the face on the masseter	Orbicularis oris at corners of mouth	Buccal branch of cranial nerve VII (facial nerve)	Retracts lips
Buccinator	Outer surfaces of mandible and maxilla	Orbicularis oris at corners of mouth	Buccal branch of cranial nerve VII (facial nerve)	Retracts lips; compresses cheeks inward
Levator labii superioris	Upper ridge of the maxilla	Middle and sides of the upper lip	Buccal branches of cranial nerve VII (facial nerve)	Elevates upper lip
Zygomatic minor	Cheekbone	Middle and sides of upper lip	Buccal branches of cranial nerve VII (facial nerve)	Elevates upper lip
Levator labii superioris alaeque nasi	On front of maxilla	Middle and sides of upper lip	Buccal branches of cranial nerve VII (facial nerve)	Elevates upper lip
Levator anguli oris	Near the canine tooth socket of the maxilla	Corners of upper and lower lips	Superior buccal branches of cranial nerve VII (facial nerve)	Pulls corners of mouth upward
Zygomatic major	Cheekbone	Corner of orbicularis oris	Buccal branches of cranial nerve VII (facial nerve)	Elevates and retracts lips
Depressor labii inferioris	Lateral surface of mandible	Lower lip	Mandibular marginal branch of cranial nerve VII (facial nerve)	Pulls lips down and out
Depressor anguli oris	Lateral mandible	Orbicularis oris, upper corner of lip	Mandibular marginal branch of cranial nerve VII (facial nerve)	Compresses upper lip; involved in producing a frown
Mentalis	Front of mandible at the level of the teeth	Skin of the chin	Mandibular marginal branch of cranial nerve VII (facial nerve)	Wrinkles chin
Platysma	Fascia covering upper chest	Corner of mouth, lower border of mandible	Cervical branch of cranial nerve VII (facial nerve)	Depresses mandible; draws mouth downward

TABLE 2-2
MUSCLES OF THE TONGUE

MUSCLE	ORIGIN	INSERTION	INNERVATION	FUNCTION
Muscles of the Tongue–Intrinsic (Innermost Muscles That Change the Shape of the Tongue)				
Superior longitudinal	Submucosal layer near *epiglottis*, hyoid, and middle vertical plane of tongue	Sides of tongue and tip of tongue	Cranial nerve XII (hypoglossal nerve)	Lifts tip of tongue; pulls tongue backward; moves tongue tip side-to-side
Inferior longitudinal	Base of tongue and hyoid bone	Tip of tongue	Cranial nerve XII (hypoglossal nerve)	Pulls tongue tip down; pulls tongue backward; moves tongue from side-to-side
Transverse	Middle vertical plane of tongue	Sides of tongue	Cranial nerve XII (hypoglossal nerve)	Narrows the tongue
Vertical	Tongue base	Membranous cover	Cranial nerve XII (hypoglossal nerve)	Pulls tongue blade downward toward the floor of the mouth; narrows tongue for protrusion
Muscles of the Tongue–Extrinsic (Outermost Muscles That Move the Tongue)				
Genioglossus	Midline of mandible	Tongue tip, surface, and body of the hyoid bone	Cranial nerve XII (hypoglossal nerve)	Pulls tongue backward (front fibers); sticks tongue out (back fibers); pulls tongue downward (front and back fibers)
Hyoglossus	Anterior midline of neck	Sides of tongue, lower longitudinal muscles	Cranial nerve XII (hypoglossal nerve)	Pulls sides of tongue downward
Styloglossus	Posterior to mandible just below the ear	Bottom sides of tongue	Cranial nerve XII (hypoglossal nerve)	Pulls tongue upward and backward into pharyngeal cavity

(continued)

TABLE 2-2 (CONTINUED)				
MUSCLES OF THE TONGUE				
MUSCLE	ORIGIN	INSERTION	INNERVATION	FUNCTION
Chondroglossus	Anterior midline of neck	Intrinsic muscles of tongue	Cranial nerve XII (hypoglossal nerve)	Depresses the tongue
Palatoglossus	Posterior border of hard palate	Sides of the back of tongue	Pharyngeal plexus from cranial nerve XI (accessory nerve) and cranial nerve X (vagus nerve)	Raises back of tongue or pulls velum down; makes up anterior faucial pillars

For example, to produce the "l" sound, the sides of the tongue must be relaxed while the tongue elevates and extends to contact the front alveolar ridge. This intricate movement involves the superior longitudinal and transverse muscles (intrinsic muscles) and the genioglossus (an extrinsic muscle) bringing the tongue forward, raising its tip, and pulling its sides away from the gums, respectively.

Swallowing requires side-to-side, in-and-out, and up-and-down movements of the tongue. Side-to-side movements enable the formation of a food bolus during chewing and clearing of the buccal cavities of debris. As food moves toward the back of the mouth, the intrinsic tongue muscles form a channel, pressing the food against the hard palate. Next, the extrinsic tongue muscles, including the genioglossus, styloglossus, and hyoglossus muscles (Figure 2-2), raise the back of the tongue and drive the bolus downward into the pharynx and, eventually, the esophagus. Because speech and swallowing rely heavily on the coordination of intricate tongue movements and a baseline level of lingual (tongue) strength, deviations in either of them can result in slurred speech and/or poor oral control of foods and liquids (see Table 2-2 for further details about major muscles of the tongue).

Another movable articulator, similar to the tongue, is the mandible. In particular, the mandible makes slight movements to assist the bottom lip, teeth, and tongue in quick and coordinated movements for speech and swallowing. The digastricus, mylohyoid, geniohyoid, and lateral pterygoid (Figure 2-3) are muscles that lower the mandible, whereas the muscles that raise the mandible include the temporalis, masseter, and medial pterygoid (Figure 2-4). These jaw depressors contain muscle spindles that are important for jaw proprioception and enable quick adjustments during speech. In addition, these depressors facilitate side-to-side, forward, and backward mandible movements simultaneously. This type of movement is facilitated by the brainstem, which signals for rhythmic contractions and a rotary grinding motion that shreds food. With the assistance of the tongue and the production of saliva via the parotid, submandibular, and sublingual salivary glands, the food may be formed into a bolus and then swallowed (see Table 2-3 for further details about major muscles of the mandible).

Unlike the tongue, lips, and mandible, the soft palate or velum (see Figure 2-1) plays the most central role in regulating whether a speech sound resonates through the mouth or nose. It also prevents food and liquids from entering the nasal cavity during swallowing by way of the velopharyngeal port (the passageway between the oral and nasal cavities). The velum accomplishes these two functions by closing the port with the levator veli palatini muscle (Figure 2-5). Specifically, the levator veli palatini raises the velum toward the back wall of the pharynx at an angle of approximately 45 degrees to prevent food, air, and speech sounds from entering the nose. To close

TABLE 2-3				
MUSCLES OF THE MANDIBLE				
MUSCLE	**ORIGIN**	**INSERTION**	**INNERVATION**	**FUNCTION**
Masseter	Cheekbone	Mandible	Anterior trunk of mandibular nerve of cranial nerve V (trigeminal nerve)	Lifts mandible
Temporalis muscle	Temporal and parietal bones of skull	Mandible	Temporal branches of mandibular nerve of cranial nerve V (trigeminal nerve)	Raises and pulls back mandible
Medial pterygoid muscle	Middle of the skull	Mandible	Mandibular branch of cranial nerve V (trigeminal nerve)	Raises mandible
Lateral pterygoid muscle	Middle of skull	Mandible	Mandibular branch of cranial nerve V (trigeminal nerve)	Protrudes mandible
Digastricus muscle (anterior)	Mandible	Anterior midline of neck	Mandibular branch of cranial nerve V (trigeminal nerve)	Pulls hyoid bone forward; lowers mandible with digastricus posterior
Digastricus muscle (posterior)	Bony prominence behind ear	Anterior midline of neck	Digastric branch of cranial nerve VII (facial nerve)	Pulls hyoid bone backward; lowers mandible with digastric anterior
Mylohyoid muscle	Mandible	Anterior midline of neck	Alveolar nerve from mandibular branch of cranial nerve V (trigeminal nerve)	Lowers mandible
Geniohyoid muscle	Mandible	Anterior mid-line of neck	Cranial nerve XII (hypoglossal nerve)	Lowers mandible
Platysma (as noted with muscles of the face)	Upper-chest muscles	Corner of mouth, lower part of mandible, near masseter	Cervical branch of cranial nerve VII (facial nerve)	Depresses mandible

this velopharyngeal port even more tightly, the musculus uvulae and the superior pharyngeal constrictor muscle (see Figure 2-5) of the pharynx will pull the back wall and sides of the pharynx forward toward the velum. During speech, the velum will typically lower only during the production of nasal speech sounds ("m, n, ng"). If the velum remains open for sounds other than "m, n, ng," a hypernasal sound quality may result and affect speech intelligibility.

During eating, the swallow is triggered reflexively after food or liquid makes contact with the velum or, in some cases, the back of the tongue or fauces. Once the swallow is triggered, the velum

TABLE 2-4				
MUSCLES OF THE VELUM				
MUSCLE	**ORIGIN**	**INSERTION**	**INNERVATION**	**FUNCTION**
Levator veli pala-tini (levator palati)	Temporal bone of skull	Posterior border of hard palate to soft palate	Pharyngeal plexus from cranial nerve XI (accessory nerve) and cranial nerve X (vagus nerve)	Raises and retracts posterior velum
Musculus uvulae	Posterior nasal cavity and posterior border of hard palate	Mucosal membrane of velum	Pharyngeal plexus from cranial nerve XI (accessory nerve) and cranial nerve X (vagus nerve)	Shortens velum
Tensor veli palatini	Bones of inner skull	Posterior border of hard palate	Mandibular nerve of cranial nerve V (trigeminal nerve)	Dilates eustachian tube
Palatoglossus	Front and side posterior bor-ders of hard palate	Sides of the back of tongue	Pharyngeal plexus from cranial nerve XI (accessory nerve) and cranial nerve X (vagus nerve)	Raises back of tongue; lowers velum; makes up anterior faucial pillars
Palatopharyngeus	Front of hard palate and middle of velum	Back portion of thyroid cartilage	Pharyngeal plexus from cranial nerve XI (accessory nerve) and cranial nerve X (vagus nerve)	Narrows walls of pharynx and low-ers velum; makes up posterior faucial pillars

closes simultaneously with the posterior fauces moving inward, the lips seal, and the tongue rises and moves posteriorly. These actions create a very brief moment of reflexive apnea (a break in respiration), which enables food to be safely moved into the esophagus without entering the nose (see Table 2-4 for further details about major muscles of the velum).

Furthest downstream from the oral cavity, lips, mandible, and velum is the pharynx. Each section of the pharynx (i.e., oropharynx, nasopharynx, and laryngopharynx) can be constricted or expanded, which affects both the quality and the type of sounds produced for speech and the propulsion of food and liquids into the esophagus. The superior, middle, and inferior constrictor muscles are responsible for making these changes to the shape of the pharynx. Specifically, the superior constrictor reduces the diameter of the oropharyngeal region, whereas the middle and inferior constrictors narrow the laryngopharyngeal region. The constrictors compress food and liquid to drive them toward the esophagus. At the base of the pharynx (i.e., upper esopha-geal sphincter) is the cricopharyngeus muscle, which relaxes to allow food into the esophagus. Figure 2-6 illustrates the complex muscle system of the pharynx. Also, see Table 2-5 for further details about major muscles of the pharynx.

TABLE 2-5				
MUSCLES OF THE PHARYNX				
MUSCLE	**ORIGIN**	**INSERTION**	**INNERVATION**	**FUNCTION**
Superior pharyngeal constrictor	Posterior mandibular angle	Pharyngeal wall	Cranial nerve X (vagus nerve) and cranial nerve XI (accessory nerve) by way of pharyngeal plexus	Brings pharyngeal wall forward and constricts walls of pharynx for swallowing
Medial pharyngeal constrictor	Anterior midline of neck and posterior to mandible behind the ear	Pharyngeal wall	Cranial nerve X (vagus nerve) and cranial nerve XI (accessory nerve) by way of pharyngeal plexus	Constricts walls of pharynx for swallowing
Inferior Pharyngeal Constrictors				
Cricopharyngeal muscle	Cricoid cartilage	Opening of esophagus	Cranial nerve X (vagus nerve) and cranial nerve XI (accessory nerve) by way of pharyngeal plexus	Constricts outer opening of esophagus for swallowing
Thyropharyngeus muscle	Thyroid cartilage	Pharyngeal wall	Cranial nerve X (vagus nerve) and cranial nerve XI (accessory nerve) by way of pharyngeal plexus	Constricts lower pharynx for swallowing
Salpingopharyngeus muscle	Lower edge of eustachian tube	Meets with palatopharyngeus muscle	Cranial nerve X (vagus nerve) and cranial nerve XI (accessory nerve) via pharyngeal plexus	Raises sides of pharyngeal wall for swallowing
Stylopharyngeus muscle	Posterior to mandible behind the ear	Into pharyngeal constrictors and back of the thyroid cartilage	Muscular branch of cranial nerve IX (glossopharyngeal nerve)	Raises and opens pharynx for swallowing

Box 2-1

Three-dimensional videos of the oral-motor, laryngeal, and respiratory anatomy are available at http://anatomyzone.com/. For video representations particularly relevant to the anatomy in question, the reader is directed to the respiratory and digestive system tutorials provided by this website.

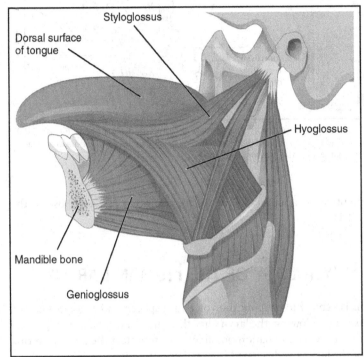

Figure 2-2. Extrinsic tongue muscles. (Reprinted with permission from http://oerpub.github.io/epubjs-demo-book/content/m46484.xhtml; it should be attributed to the following based on Wikimedia commons: by OpenStax College [CC BY 3.0 (http://creativecommons.org/licenses/by/3.0)], via Wikimedia Commons.)

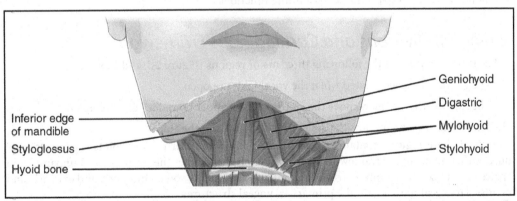

Figure 2-3. Muscles that lower the mandible. (Reprinted with permission from OpenStax College [CC BY 3.0 (http://creativecommons.org/licenses/by/3.0)], via Wikimedia Commons at https://upload.wikimedia.org/wikipedia/commons/7/74/1110_Muscle_of_the_Anterior_Neck.jpg.)

At this point, it should be noted that the structures of the oral-motor system do not perform isolated functions. Rather, they are integrated collectively and coordinated for speech and swallowing. As mentioned previously, the mandible assists in articulation of the lips, tongue, and teeth. Also, the tongue, fauces, velum, and pharynx work together for moving food back and

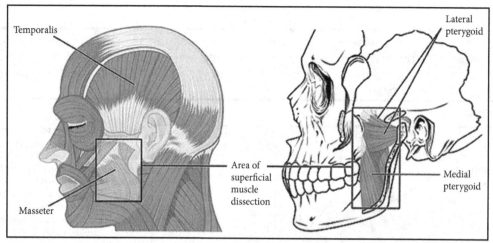

Figure 2-4. Muscles that raise the mandible. (Reprinted with permission from OpenStax College [CC BY 3.0 (http://creativecommons.org/licenses/by/3.0)], via Wikimedia Commons at https://upload.wikimedia.org/wikipedia/commons/3/30/1108_Muscle_that_Move_the_Lower_Jaw.jpg.)

downward. The muscle movements and functions of each structure often rely on those of the adjacent structures (Case Study 2-1).

ANATOMY AND PHYSIOLOGY OF THE HUMAN LARYNX

While the oral-motor system is central to shaping the voice into speech and is important for chewing and the beginning phase of swallowing, the larynx has three main purposes: to help regulate airflow to and from the lungs, to make phonation possible, and to protect the airway. In this section, the complex anatomy of the larynx is discussed in detail and functionally linked to these communicative, protective, and life-sustaining functions.

Laryngeal Divisions and Cartilaginous Framework

The larynx consists of the following three major regions (Figure 2-7 and Box 2-2):

1. The *glottis*, the space created when the vocal folds are open

2. The *supraglottis*, the area above the glottis with its upper boundary at the epiglottis

3. The *subglottis*, which spans the area below the glottis to the trachea

Each of these regions contains a variety of cartilaginous structures, joints, ligaments, and muscles that make up the framework of the larynx. In particular, the hyoid bone, 3 unpaired and 3 paired cartilages, two joints, extrinsic and intrinsic ligaments and membranes, and extrinsic and intrinsic laryngeal muscles are the primary laryngeal structures.

Hyoid Bone

Although not technically a structure of the larynx, the hyoid bone is often considered part of the laryngeal framework simply because the entire larynx is suspended from it. Shaped like a horseshoe, the hyoid bone lies toward the anterior neck at midline, just below the chin (Figure 2-8). Unlike other bones, the hyoid does not attach directly to any other bone in the body. Rather, ligaments, membranes, and muscles stabilize and allow for movement and suspension of the larynx from the hyoid bone.

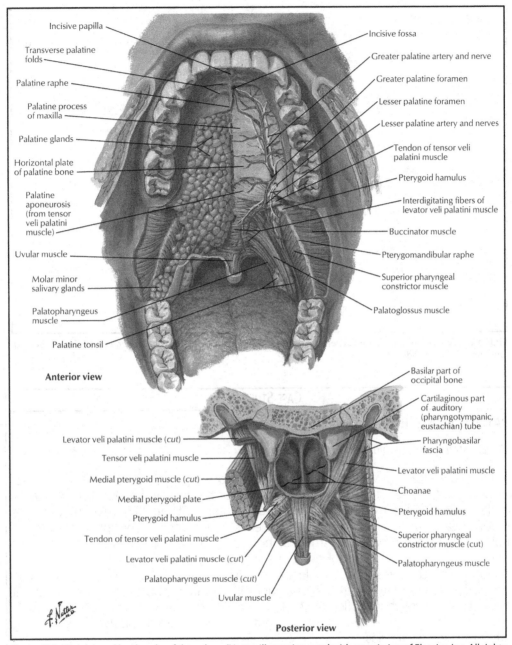

Figure 2-5. Muscles and landmarks of the velum. (Netter illustration used with permission of Elsevier, Inc. All rights reserved. www.netterimages.com.)

Laryngeal Cartilages

The following cartilages support the larynx and form its skeleton:

- The epiglottis is a leaf-shaped cartilage situated in the supraglottic region of the larynx behind the hyoid bone and at the root of the tongue (Figure 2-9). Its top is broad, round, and thin and narrows into a stalk-like structure toward the bottom. Although the epiglottis does not contribute significantly to speech, it folds backward to cover and protect the airway during

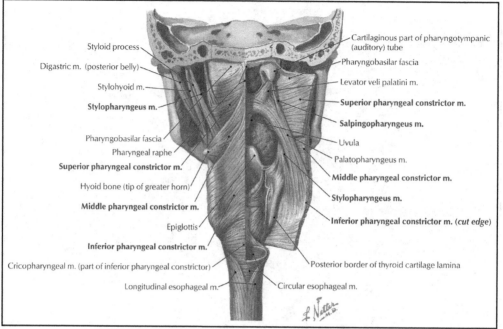

Figure 2-6. Muscles of the pharynx. (Netter illustration used with permission of Elsevier, Inc. All rights reserved. www.netterimages.com.)

CASE STUDY 2-1

PATIENT NAME: ROBIN

Clinical Status: initial evaluation for suspected LC

Robin, a 62-year-old woman, presented to the otolaryngologist complaining of hoarseness, shortness of breath, and trouble swallowing that had worsened over a 6-month period. Her previous medical history included chronic obstructive pulmonary disease (COPD), treated with daily *corticosteroid* inhaler use, and chronic laryngopharyngeal reflux. Robin stated that although she smoked about one pack of cigarettes per day for more than 20 years, she had quit smoking approximately 3 years ago. She actively worked as a customer service representative and reported that she recently had difficulty projecting her voice. Robin frequently experienced difficulty breathing because of her COPD but noted that her breathing difficulties had increased in severity over the previous month. She denied blood in her sputum and weight loss. She reported coughing and choking when drinking thin liquids.

Visualization of the larynx with a rigid *endoscope* identified a large white lesion on Robin's right true vocal fold. Her right vocal fold was also fixed in position. The irregular anatomy of the right true vocal fold resulted in impaired vocal fold vibration with incomplete vocal fold closure and compensatory ventricular vocal fold activity. Perceptually, her voice was severely rough and breathy because of the impaired vibration and movement of the right vocal fold that resulted from the mass. Robin also exhibited a limited ability to produce variation in pitch and loudness or sustain phonation. A computerized tomography scan revealed other masses on the epiglottis (supraglottically) and within the trachea (subglottically). Biopsy of the lesions revealed a squamous cell carcinoma that had grown

(continued)

CASE STUDY 2-1 (CONTINUED)

into body tissue outside the larynx (T4). Robin's symptoms of dyspnea were likely related to the presence of the carcinoma in the subglottic airway. In addition, her coughing when ingesting thin liquids was likely a result of compromised airway protection, because the right vocal fold was unable to contact the left vocal fold during swallowing, and movement of the ventricular folds and epiglottis was restricted because of the location of the supraglottic masses. The sensation of a lump in the throat described by Robin may indeed have been related to her sensing the masses on, below, and above her vocal folds. Robin was referred immediately to a LC care team at a regional medical center for treatment planning and implementation.

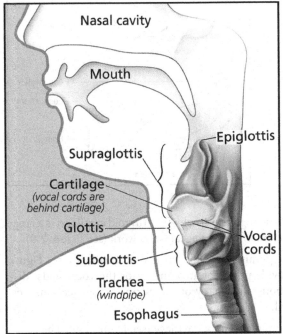

Figure 2-7. Lateral view of the head and neck showing regions of the larynx and the relationship of the larynx to the head, trachea, and esophagus. (Reprinted with permission from Alan Hoofring [illustrator] [public domain], via Wikimedia Commons at https:// upload.wikimedia.org/wikipedia/commons/b/b2/ Larynx_and_nearby_structures.jpg)

BOX 2-2

For animations and additional views of the larynx, the reader is referred to the *Interactive Atlas of the Larynx* by Ahmet Sinav, MD: https://www1.columbia.edu/sec/itc/hs/medical/ anatomy_resources/anatomy/larynx/.

swallowing. In addition, to preserve this important function, the epiglottis does not harden like other laryngeal cartilages across the lifespan (Noordzij & Ossoff, 2006).

- Spanning the subglottic, supraglottic, and glottic regions of the larynx is the thyroid cartilage. Thyroid is Latin for shield, which is an indication of the protection it provides to the larynx against trauma (see Figure 2-9). Likewise, similar to a shield, the thyroid cartilage spans the sides and the front of the larynx only and is open in the back. Important landmarks of this cartilage include the thyroid notch and thyroid prominence, which is commonly referred to as the Adam's apple.

Figure 2-8. Position of the hyoid bone in the neck and its associated features on anterior and right lateral views. (Reprinted with permission from OpenStax College [CC BY 3.0 (http://creativecommons.org/licenses/by/3.0)], via Wikimedia Commons at https://upload.wikimedia.org/wikipedia/commons/8/83/712_Hyoid_Bone.jpg.)

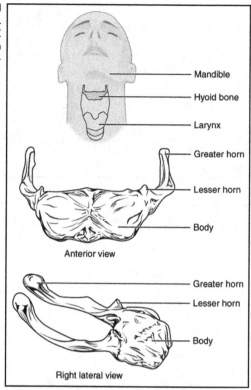

- The cricoid cartilage, located in the subglottic region and below the thyroid cartilage, is a ring-shaped structure that forms the lower portion of the laryngeal framework (see Figure 2-9).

- On the back of the cricoid cartilage sit the pyramidal-shaped arytenoid cartilages (see Figure 2-9). The paired arytenoid cartilages provide points of attachment for the vocal folds (discussed in more detail in subsequent sections) and many of the intrinsic laryngeal muscles, which pull the vocal folds open and closed.

- Positioned atop each arytenoid cartilage is a corniculate cartilage (see Figure 2-9). The cone-shaped corniculate cartilages may be thought of as extensions of the arytenoid cartilages and may possibly assist with opening and closing the vocal folds by providing better attachment points for laryngeal musculature.

- The cuneiform cartilages are a pair of wedge-shaped rods imbedded within connective tissue, fat, and mucous membrane that are referred to collectively as the aryepiglottic folds (Figure 2-10). The cuneiform cartilages lend support to the aryepiglottic folds and stiffen them to help maintain a patent opening to the larynx.

Vocal, Aryepiglottic, and Ventricular Folds

Many of the structures that are protected or supported by the cartilages already discussed are a series of folds of tissues that are central to airway protection and phonation. Linking the epiglottis with the arytenoids are the aryepiglottic folds, which also contain the aryepiglottic muscle responsible for folding the epiglottis (i.e., pulling it back and down) over the laryngeal opening to divert food into the esophagus. Also during swallowing, the ventricular folds, located inferior to the aryepiglottic folds and superior to the vocal folds, may meet at midline to close and prevent food and liquids from entering the airway when the epiglottis has failed to prevent materials from

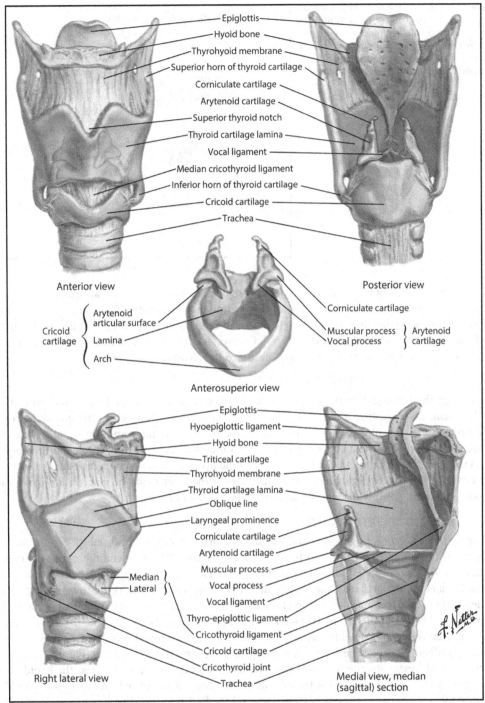

Figure 2-9. Laryngeal cartilages and component parts. (Netter illustration used with permission of Elsevier, Inc. All rights reserved. www.netterimages.com.)

moving below it. In some cases, the ventricular folds are vibrated against one another and used as a voicing source instead of the vocal folds. Ventricular phonation may occur when the vocal folds are injured or there is excessive muscle tension that results in poorly coordinated phonation. The vocal folds are of utmost interest to those who study the larynx and the conditions that affect it, such

Figure 2-10. Superior view of the larynx, including the vocal, aryepiglottic, and ventricular folds. (Reprinted with permission from Henry Vandyke Carter [public domain], via Wikimedia Commons at https://upload.wikimedia.org/wikipedia/commons/b/bd/Gray1204.png.)

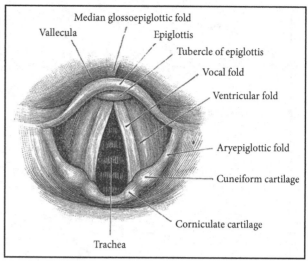

as LC. They are folds of bilateral tissue with a complex layer structure that affords them unique vibratory properties for phonation (Hirano, 1974). Similar to the ventricular folds, the vocal folds also close during swallowing, which provides a third layer of protection against airway invasion (see Figure 2-10 for visuals of these structures). Greater detail about the roles of these structures in phonation, respiration, and swallowing are discussed in subsequent sections.

Laryngeal Ligaments and Membranes

Although the laryngeal cartilages provide a primary structure for the larynx and protection for the vocal, aryepiglottic, and ventricular folds, connections between cartilages are formed by ligaments (e.g., thyrohyoid ligaments connect the thyroid cartilage and the hyoid bone), and the spaces between these cartilages are filled in via membranes (e.g., the thyrohyoid membrane covers the space between the thyroid cartilage and the hyoid bone, creating a tube-like structure). Collectively, the laryngeal ligaments and membranes of the larynx may be placed into one of two categories: extrinsic or intrinsic laryngeal ligaments and membranes.

Extrinsic Ligaments and Membranes

The extrinsic laryngeal ligaments and membranes provide support and stability to the larynx by connecting structures within it to those outside it. Many of these membranes and ligaments connect the laryngeal cartilages to the hyoid bone, which, as previously noted, is the suspension site for the larynx. In particular, the middle thyrohyoid ligament connects the thyroid notch (i.e., the depression at the top-middle portion of the thyroid cartilage) to the bottom of the middle of the anterior hyoid bone. Similarly, the two lateral thyrohyoid ligaments connect the thyroid cartilage to the open ends of each side of the hyoid bone. Finally, the thyrohyoid membrane covers the ligaments and fills in the space between the thyroid cartilage and the hyoid bone (Figure 2-11). Like the thyrohyoid ligaments, the hyoepiglottic ligament connects the epiglottis and the hyoid bone (see Figure 2-11). Also similar to the thyrohyoid membrane, the cricotracheal membrane provides coverage for space between the cricoid cartilage and the first tracheal ring.

Intrinsic Ligaments and Membranes

The extrinsic ligaments and membranes are supportive and structural in nature, whereas the intrinsic ligaments and membranes serve to connect laryngeal cartilages with each other to regulate movements within the laryngeal apparatus. Connecting all structures with one another (i.e., the thyroid, cricoid, and arytenoids; Zemlin, 1998) and filling all of the subglottic space, the conus elasticus comprises the medial cricothyroid ligament and two lateral cricothyroid membranes

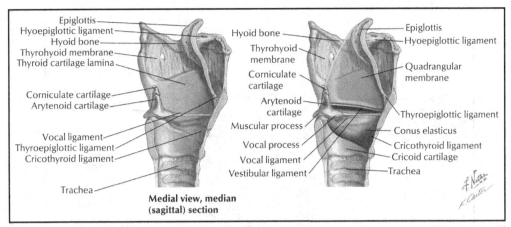

Figure 2-11. Laryngeal membranes and ligaments. (Netter illustration used with permission of Elsevier, Inc. All rights reserved. www.netterimages.com.)

(see Figure 2-11). The cricothyroid ligaments, as their name suggests, connects the cricoid cartilage with the bottom border of the thyroid angle (see Figure 2-11). The two lateral cricothyroid membranes span the top border of the cricoid cartilage to the undersides of the arytenoid cartilages and to the bottom-middle part of the thyroid cartilage. The free borders of the conus elasticus form the vocal folds.

The quadrangular membranes are paired and connect the supraglottic structures and fill all space from the top of the larynx down to the level of the vocal folds (see Figure 2-11). Specifically, the quadrangular membranes connect the epiglottis with the arytenoid and thyroid cartilages and form the false vocal folds inferiorly and the aryepiglottic folds superiorly. Finally, mucous membrane lines the mouth and extends to the pharynx and down through the larynx and trachea. It adheres closely to the epiglottis, aryepiglottic folds, and vocal folds and is especially rich in mucous glands within the ventricle (space) between the true and false vocal folds.

Laryngeal Joints

Laryngeal joints, including the cricoarytenoid and cricothyroid joints, enable laryngeal cartilages to move against one another, alter the length of laryngeal ligaments, and change the configuration of the vocal folds. Formed at the juncture of each of the arytenoid cartilages and the areas of the cricoid cartilage on which they sit, the cricoarytenoid joints enable the arytenoid cartilages to rotate or rock when the attached intrinsic laryngeal muscles (detailed later) contract. This action allows the vocal folds to open for respiration and close for phonation and airway protection.

The cricothyroid joints are formed at the junction of the cricoid cartilage and the inferior thyroid horns (see Figures 2-9 and 2-14). The cricothyroid joints allow rotational and some gliding movements when the cricothyroid muscle contracts, which, in turn, lengthens and tenses the vocal folds to increase vocal pitch.

Laryngeal Muscles

The muscles of the larynx play a central role in facilitating vocal fold movement (i.e., intrinsic laryngeal muscles) and in the function of the larynx as a whole (i.e., extrinsic laryngeal muscles). Similar to the ligaments, membranes, and joints previously discussed, muscles of the larynx also may be grouped into categories on the basis of their points of attachment (i.e., whether they connect with structures only within the larynx or connect structures within the larynx to those outside it).

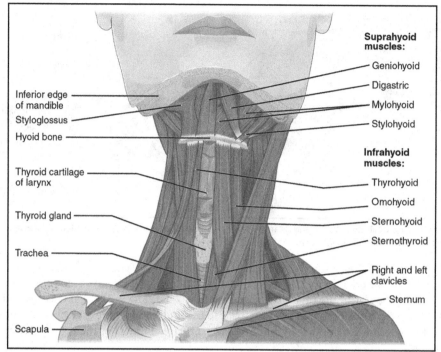

Figure 2-12. Extrinsic muscles, including the suprahyoid (above the hyoid bone) and infrahyoid (below the hyoid bone) muscles. (Reprinted with permission from OpenStax College [CC BY 3.0 (http://creativecommons.org/licenses/by/3.0)], via Wikimedia Commons at https://upload.wikimedia.org/wikipedia/commons/7/74/1110_Muscle_of_the_Anterior_Neck.jpg.)

Extrinsic Muscles

Extrinsic laryngeal muscles enable movement of the larynx (e.g., raising and lowering) and provide support through stabilization of the larynx. Typically, the extrinsic laryngeal muscles are discussed relative to their position with the hyoid bone and include the suprahyoid (above the hyoid bond) and infrahyoid (below the hyoid bone) muscle groups.

The suprahyoid muscle group consists of the extrinsic laryngeal muscles that are attached to the hyoid bone and a structure above it. These muscles include the stylohyoid, mylohyoid, geniohyoid, and digastric muscles (Figure 2-12). In general, when these muscles contract, the hyoid and suspended larynx move upward and forward, an action important for swallowing, because this movement protects the airway and allows food and/or liquid to enter the esophagus. Because these muscles elevate the hyoid bone, they are also often referred to as laryngeal elevators. These muscles were also previously discussed in relation to the oral-motor system, because they also function as jaw depressors.

The infrahyoid muscle group consists of the extrinsic laryngeal muscles that are attached to the hyoid bone and a structure below it and include the omohyoid, sternohyoid, thyrohyoid, and sternothyroid muscles (see Figure 2-12). In general, when these muscles contract, the hyoid and suspended larynx lower. Because these muscles depress the hyoid bone, they are often referred to as laryngeal depressors.

Intrinsic Muscles

Largely responsible for the control of sound production and respiratory valving, the intrinsic laryngeal muscles include the thyroarytenoid (TA), posterior cricoarytenoid (PCA), lateral cricoarytenoid (LCA), interarytenoid, and cricothyroid (CT) muscles (Figures 2-13 and 2-14). These muscles may be grouped according to how they affect the shape of the glottis. During quiet

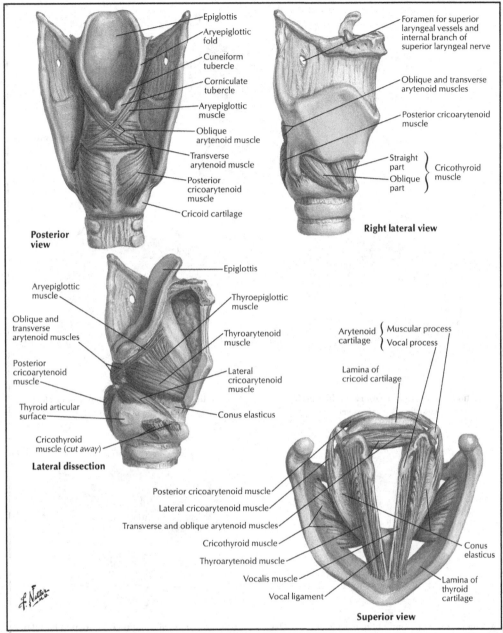

Figure 2-13. Intrinsic muscles of the larynx. (Netter illustration used with permission of Elsevier, Inc. All rights reserved. www.netterimages.com.)

breathing, the glottis is wide open because the vocal folds are in an abducted (i.e., open) position. The intrinsic laryngeal muscles that make abduction possible are the paired PCA muscles. The paired LCA, TA, and interarytenoid muscles contribute to adducting (i.e., bringing together) the vocal folds, and the LCAs are the primary muscles of adduction. The act of adducting the vocal folds makes voicing possible, and the actual closing of the vocal folds is another measure of protection for the airway during swallowing, as was indicated previously. The LCA muscle has many rapidly contracting muscle fibers that subserve this role (Shiotani, Westra, & Flint, 1999; Wu, Crumley, Armstrong, & Caiozzo, 2000). The CT, when contracted, tenses or lengthens the vocal

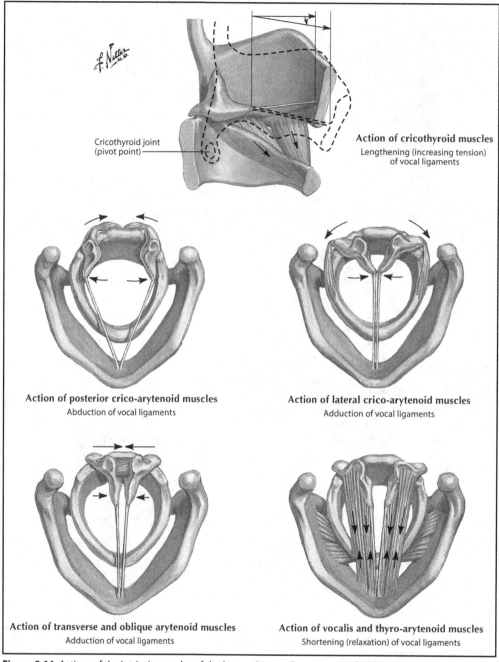

Action of cricothyroid muscles
Lengthening (increasing tension)
of vocal ligaments

Cricothyroid joint
(pivot point)

Action of posterior crico-arytenoid muscles
Abduction of vocal ligaments

Action of lateral crico-arytenoid muscles
Adduction of vocal ligaments

Action of transverse and oblique arytenoid muscles
Adduction of vocal ligaments

Action of vocalis and thyro-arytenoid muscles
Shortening (relaxation) of vocal ligaments

Figure 2-14. Actions of the intrinsic muscles of the larynx. (Netter illustration used with permission of Elsevier, Inc. All rights reserved. www.netterimages.com.)

folds, which results in an increase in vocal pitch (Noordzij & Ossoff, 2006; Shipp, 1975). In contrast, during low-pitch phonation, contraction of the TA muscles occurs to shorten the vocal folds. Although the CT and TA muscles may be activated in combination to produce changes in pitch, at extremely low pitches, there will be little to no activation of the CT and maximal activation of the TA, and at extremely high pitches, there will be little to no activation of the TA muscle and maximal activation of the CT muscle (Shipp, 1975). Of all the intrinsic muscles, the TA muscle is the only one that is actually a part of the true vocal folds. All the others are connected to the cartilages for which they are named to manipulate the distance from one cartilage to another, which, in turn, affects the length, tension, and adduction/abduction of the vocal folds.

Laryngeal Innervation

The vagus nerve (cranial nerve X) is typically considered the primary source of sensory and motor innervation to the larynx (Zemlin, 1998). Latin for wanderer, the vagus nerve extends from the brainstem to each side of the neck, coursing between the internal jugular vein and the internal carotid artery. On both the right and left sides of the neck, the vagus branches into the superior laryngeal nerve (SLN) and the recurrent laryngeal nerve (RLN) (Figure 2-15).

The SLN branches high in the neck from the main trunk of the vagus nerve and, in turn, sub-divides into two parts: the internal laryngeal branch and the external laryngeal branch. Inserting into the left and right sides of the thyrohyoid membrane, the internal laryngeal branch provides sensory innervation to the mucous membrane as far down as the vocal folds and their adjacent areas. The internal laryngeal branch warns the brain that something has gone down the "wrong pipe." This warning can lead to the essential triggering of a cough and expulsion of the invading material. The external laryngeal branch provides motor innervation to the right and left sides of the cricothyroid muscle to facilitate increases in vocal pitch.

The RLN branches lower in the neck from the main trunk of cranial nerve X, with the right RLN looping around the subclavian artery just below the collarbone and traveling up to the larynx and the left RLN looping around the aorta near the heart and traveling up to the larynx. The RLN provides motor innervation to all of the intrinsic laryngeal muscles except the cricothyroid muscle, which is innervated by the external laryngeal branch of the SLN. Trauma to the RLN (i.e., surgical, accidental, etc.) may result in paralysis of one (unilateral) or both (bilateral) vocal folds.

Laryngeal Functions

As stated previously, the larynx serves three functions; it regulates airflow in and out of the lungs, it protects the airway, and it makes phonation possible. Although these functions are discussed briefly throughout this chapter, additional details about these functions are provided here.

Regulating Airflow

The larynx provides a passageway for oxygen to flow into the trachea. In fact, without abduction of the vocal folds, respiration would not be possible. The larynx is also able to alter its resistance to airflow and, in turn, regulate the amount of air that flows in and out of the vocal folds (Kuna, Insalaco, & Woodson, 1988). Observations of the larynx during respiration have revealed that the glottis widens on inhalation and narrows slightly on exhalation. The degrees of this widening and narrowing vary according to how much airflow is required. For example, respiratory demand is greater when the body is moving versus when it is at rest. Likewise, respiratory demand is greater during communicative activities, such as singing and yelling vs quiet talking. In addition to the movement of the glottis, the true vocal folds function as a valving mechanism that opens for quiet breathing and closes for speech, swallowing, and other actions that require increased subglottal pressure (e.g., coughing).

In some disease processes and disorders of the larynx and even with normal laryngeal aging, weakening or even paralysis of one or both vocal folds may prevent them from closing firmly. When this occurs, air escapes through the glottis and prevents subglottic pressure from effectively building below the vocal folds, which results in a weak and breathy voice and a weak cough when expulsion of materials is needed. Vocal fold tumors often cause hoarseness or other changes in the voice. If allowed to grow, the tumor will intrude on the airway and make breathing more difficult. In normal aging, the body loses muscle mass through a physiological process called atrophy. Because the true vocal folds contain muscles (e.g., the TA muscle), they often atrophy as part of the normal aging process. A possible consequence of vocal fold atrophy is an inability for the folds to close firmly. Again, when the true vocal folds cannot close firmly, subglottic pressure cannot build, yielding a voice that, in part, sounds breathy and lower in volume.

Figure 2-15. Innervation of the larynx. (Reprinted with permission from Jkwchui [based on drawing by Truth-seeker2004] [CC BY-SA 3.0 (http://creativecommons. org/licenses/ by-sa/3.0)], via Wikimedia Commons at https://upload.wikimedia. org/wikipedia/commons/6/64/Recurrent_ laryngeal_nerve.svg.)

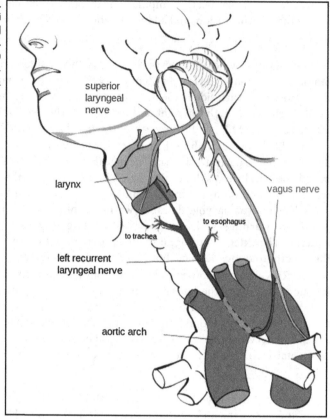

superior laryngeal nerve

larynx

vagus nerve

to esophagus

to trachea

left recurrent laryngeal nerve

aortic arch

Protection of the Airway

Because of its position above the trachea, the primary biological function of the larynx is to protect the lower airway. Anatomically, the vocal folds are situated slightly higher than and just in front of the esophagus. Because the pharynx opens into both the larynx and the esophagus, it is imperative that some biomechanical processes exist to guide food and liquid to the area behind the vocal folds so that they enter the esophagus instead of the airway. This biomechanical process is referred to as *hyolaryngeal excursion.*

In a normal swallow, hyolaryngeal excursion occurs when the suprahyoid muscles (extrinsic laryngeal muscles) contract, resulting in the upward and forward movement of the hyoid bone, and, in turn, the larynx. When these actions occur, the epiglottis folds over the glottis to cover the entrance of the airway and guide the food and/or liquid to the esophagus. Simultaneously, the aryepiglottic folds and false vocal folds stiffen and close, and, as a final layer of protection for the airway, the RLN signals the LCA, TA, and IA muscles (intrinsic laryngeal muscles) to contract in order to facilitate vocal fold adduction. This adduction subsequently halts respiration and prevents foreign material from entering the airway. Once food material has entered the esophagus and the swallow is complete, the infrahyoid muscles (extrinsic laryngeal muscles) depress the hyoid bone and larynx, which results in their return to the normal position, the unfolding of the epiglottis, and the relaxation and opening of the aryepiglottic and false vocal folds. Finally, the RLN signals the PCA muscles (intrinsic laryngeal muscles) to contract, which results in abduction of the vocal folds so that respiration can resume.

At times, foreign matter (e.g., food, saliva) may enter the larynx. When the SLN detects a foreign substance, the RLN responds by signaling the LCA, TA, and IA muscles (intrinsic laryngeal muscles) to adduct the vocal folds. As a result, respiration halts, and the substance is prevented

---

Box 2-3

Videos showing the vocal folds during phonation, respiration, and airway protective functions are provided at the following websites:

https://www.youtube.com/watch?v=VRAU33_s4ec (breathing and phonation)

https://www.youtube.com/watch?v=usAqJoVYVSc (coughing/airway protection)

https://youtu.be/l8elCovpb28 (swallowing and visualization of PE segment)

---

from entering into the airway. In addition, the cough reflex is triggered to expel the material from the larynx.

Cough strength is determined by the amount of subglottic pressure generated. Subglottic pressure, in turn, is determined by the ability of the two vocal folds to close. In some disease processes and disorders, and even with normal aging, dysfunction of the RLN or vocal fold weakness may compromise glottic closure. When this happens, air escapes through the glottis and prevents subglottic pressure from building effectively. The degree of air leakage is inversely related to cough strength (e.g., the greater the air leakage, the weaker the cough). Therefore, if the cough is weak, airway protection will be compromised.

Making Phonation Possible

For sound to occur (whether for speaking, laughing, or singing), the vocal folds must vibrate. Vibration happens when the vocal folds are close enough to the air flowing through the glottic region that the air stream causes the vocal folds to come together repeatedly (Titze, 1994; van den Berg, 1958). This approximation effectively "chops" up the airstream, such that it is no longer a continuous flow of air but rather a series of "puffs" that then excite the upper airway (i.e., cavities of the oral-motor system [Rothenberg, 1983]). This series of "puffs" is created at great speeds. For example, the average rate at which the vocal folds vibrate (open and close) is approximately 200 times/second for a woman, 100 times/seconds for a man, and 300 times/second for a child. Of course, these are average values, and acceptable ranges have been determined because vocal fold vibratory speed depends on several characteristics, including, age, body size, health, and speaking task (Hixon, Weismer, & Hoit, 2013).

In addition to sound, the larynx also manipulates pitch and volume. Innervation of the CT muscle (intrinsic laryngeal muscle) by the SLN results in the downward and forward movement of the thyroid cartilage via the cricothyroid joint. This action lengthens and stretches the two vocal folds (Box 2-3). Innervation of the TA muscle by the RLN results in decreasing the length and tension of the vocal folds, thereby lowering pitch. The larynx manipulates volume through the glottic region. To make the voice louder, subglottic pressure must be increased. Yelling, for example, requires greater subglottic pressure than speaking to someone who is only a few feet away.

ANATOMY AND PHYSIOLOGY OF HUMAN RESPIRATION

As previously indicated, the larynx provides a sound source for phonation and a means by which the vocal folds can regulate the amount of air that leaves or enters the respiratory system, and it protects the respiratory system from aspirating foods or liquids. Thus, the respiratory system depends on the actions of the larynx for protection and airway valving, and the larynx depends on the respiratory system to provide the air supply that sets the vocal folds into vibration for phonation. In addition, while the larynx, and specifically the vocal folds, is the gateway by which air is allowed into or out of the respiratory system, the gas exchange, paramount to human survival,

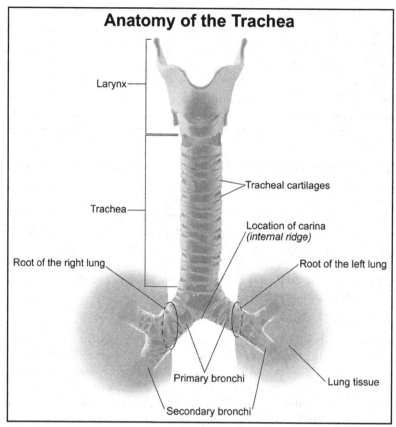

Anatomy of the Trachea

Larynx

Trachea

Tracheal cartilages

Location of carina
(internal ridge)

Root of the right lung

Root of the left lung

Primary bronchi

Lung tissue

Secondary bronchi

Figure 2-16. The trachea. (Reprinted with permission from Bruce Blaus. Blausen.com staff. "Blausen gallery 2014." Wikiversity Journal of Medicine. DOI: 10.15347/wjm/2014.010. ISSN 20018762. [Own work] [CC BY 3.0 (http://creativecommons.org/licenses/by/3.0)], via Wikimedia Commons at https://upload.wikimedia.org/wikipedia/commons/4/4c/ Blausen_0865_TracheaAnatomy.png.)

takes place downstream in this system. Thus, in this section, a brief overview of the structures of the respiratory system is provided and connected to their functional role in the respiratory process.

Trachea

Extending from the larynx to the bronchi, the trachea is composed of 16 to 20 horseshoe-shaped cartilages, open at the back, that are stacked one atop the other, separated by a fibroelastic membrane that provides protection from friction (Figure 2-16). The open area of the posterior trachea is actually closed off because of its direct contact with the esophagus. Thus, the trachea can be thought of as an 11- to 12-cm tube (Zemlin, 1998) that remains perpetually open because of the rigidity of its cartilaginous rings. The space at the back of the trachea includes fibrous tissue and smooth muscle that permits stretching, twisting, and/or compression.

The cricotracheal ligaments and membrane connect with and fill the space between the first tracheal cartilage and the bottom border of the cricoid cartilage. At the last tracheal cartilage, the trachea splits into two sections (bifurcates), giving rise to the main stem or primary bronchus. The carina, the ridge-like structure located at the point of bifurcation, is an important landmark (see Figure 2-16).

As with the laryngeal tube, the trachea is covered by a membrane. The tracheal membrane is continuous with the previously described mucous membranes that line the mouth, pharynx,

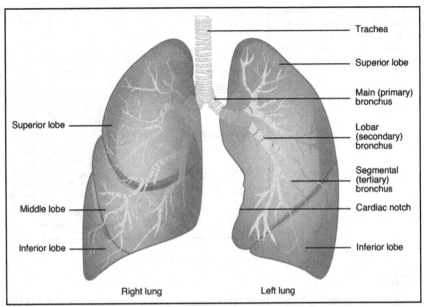

Figure 2-17. Bronchi within the lungs. (Reprinted with permission from OpenStax College [CC BY 3.0 (http://creativecommons.org/licenses/by/3.0)], via Wikimedia Commons at https://upload.wikimedia.org/wikipedia/commons/7/7e/2312_Gross_Anatomy_of_the_Lungs.jpg.)

larynx, and trachea. This membrane, referred to as the tracheal membrane because of its location, consists of two layers, one that passes over the outer surface of the cartilaginous rings and another that passes over the inner surface of the rings. These layers form the intratracheal membrane, which connects the tracheal rings with each other and traps small matter and micro-organisms via tracheal cilia (hair-like structures) that line these layers and transport mucous, smoke particles, and dust out of the lungs through their up-and-down motions.

Bronchi

Structurally similar to the trachea, the bronchi consist of two tubes that extend from the trachea to the lungs, where they form the bronchial tree (see Figures 2-16 and 2-17). In comparison to the left main stem bronchus, the right main stem bronchus is larger in diameter, is half its length, and forms more of a direct line with the trachea. Food matter and other impurities may enter into the right bronchus more easily because of its orientation to the trachea (Zemlin, 1998).

The bronchi belong to one of the three following groups:

1. The main stem bronchi connect the trachea to each lung.

2. The secondary bronchi, which are formed when the main stem bronchi divide; specifically, the right bronchus divides into three secondary bronchi, one for each lobe of the right lung, and the left bronchus divides into two secondary bronchi, one for each of the two lobes of the left lung. The right secondary bronchus subdivides into 10 tertiary bronchi, each of which supplies a segment of the right lung, and the left secondary bronchus subdivides into eight tertiary bronchi, each of which supplies a segment of the left lung.

3. The tertiary bronchi divide repeatedly from below the level of the secondary bronchi, becoming smaller and smaller until they are almost microscopic (24 divisions). The final division of tertiary bronchi gives rise to the bronchioles.

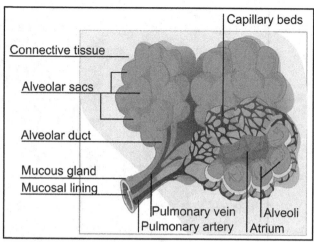

Figure 2-18. Alveoli. (Reprinted with permission from LadyofHats [public domain], via Wikimedia Commons at https://upload.wikimedia.org/wikipedia/commons/4/46/Alveolus_diagram.svg.)

Bronchioles

Bronchioles are distinguished from bronchi in that they do not contain cartilage or glands. The bronchioles are responsible for controlling air distribution and airflow resistance in the lungs. Repeated divisions ultimately give rise to terminal bronchioles, which branch to form alveolar ducts.

Alveoli

Appearing as small pockets, the alveoli form depressions in the walls of terminal bronchioles (Figure 2-18). They are the smallest and most numerous subdivisions of the respiratory system. The alveolar walls are covered in capillaries and separated from air by a thin membrane. It is remarkable that the total area in contact with a capillary bed is approximately 70 to 90 m². The thin barrier and large area support rapid exchanges of oxygen and carbon dioxide. In the alveolar ducts, alveoli appear as out-pockets (see Figure 2-18). Alveolar ducts divide into two or three alveolar sacs, in which oxygen and carbon dioxide exchange occurs.

Lungs

The site of the bronchi, bronchioles, and alveoli are the lungs. Composed of spongy, porous, and highly elastic material, the lungs are two roughly cone-shaped organs located in the thoracic cavity (see Figure 2-17). The right lung is larger, shorter, and broader than the left lung to make space for the liver, which occupies the upper right abdominal cavity and forces the dome of the diaphragm higher in the thorax. Likewise, the right lung is divided into three lobes by two fissures, and the left lung is divided into two lobes by one fissure (see Figure 2-17). The heart occupies much of the left side of the thorax, which accounts for the smaller left lung and lower number of lobes. Both the right and left lungs extend into the bottom of the neck superiorly and atop the diaphragm inferiorly. The inferior lungs are actually broad and concave to conform to the top of the diaphragm.

Pulmonary Surfactant

The lungs have a predisposition to collapse inward because of their elastic nature. Collapse is prevented by pulmonary surfactant, a lipoprotein that maintains the surface tension that is created by the attraction between the water molecules in the alveoli and provides lubrication to ease alveolar expansion. Pulmonary surfactant keeps the pulmonary tissue moist, thereby creating an air–liquid interface. As can be imagined, insufficient surfactant results in breathing problems.

BOX 2-4

For videos depicting the mechanics of the respiratory process, the reader is directed to the following videos:

https://www.youtube.com/watch?v=lr5dDmTASos

https://www.youtube.com/watch?v=hp-gCvW8PRY

Pleural Linkage

Two kinds of membranes line the thoracic cavity, the parietal/costal pleura, which covers the inner surface of the thoracic cage, and the visceral pleura, which covers the lungs following its contours. The pleurae encase the lungs, and the space between the parietal and visceral pleurae is filled with intrapleural fluid. The pleural linkage also combats the lungs' tendency toward collapse. Negative pressure between the pleural membranes holds the lungs against the thoracic wall. Negative pressure is created by absorption of intrapleural fluids by the visceral pleura and by the pull of the lungs against the thoracic wall. Throughout every breath cycle, the lung surfaces are held tightly against the inner surface of the thoracic walls. The surface tension of fluid links the lungs and thoracic cavity together, which allows the lungs and thorax to operate as one unit (Agostini & Mead, 1964).

Mechanics of Respiration

All of the structures of the respiratory system reviewed in the previous sections allow respiration to occur in the following predictable sequence (Box 2-4):

1. The diaphragm contracts and moves downward. This vertical excursion has been found to range anywhere from 1.5 to 7 cm during quiet and deep breathing, respectively (Wade & Gilson, 1951). The ribs move outward while the chest moves outward and upward. These actions cause the lungs to expand in each direction as they are linked by the pleurae to the diaphragm, ribs, and sternum.

2. This expansion, in turn, creates a negative pressure inside the lungs, which must be filled until the pressure in the lungs is equal to the pressure outside the lungs.

3. Once the lungs fill with oxygen and a positive pressure is created, the lungs expel carbon dioxide from the system through elastic recoil, and negative pressure is once again created. During quiet breathing, active muscular force is needed only on inspiration, but passive expiratory recoil can lead to air expulsion without expiratory muscle activity on expiration (Zemlin, 1998). During speech, passive recoil and respiratory muscles work together to facilitate expiration.

4. With this continuous cycle of pressure changes, the body inhales oxygen, which enters the lungs and flows to the alveoli. Oxygen then enters the bloodstream through the thin barrier between the alveoli and capillaries. During exhalation, carbon dioxide flows out of the alveoli and exits the lungs as well as the bloodstream.

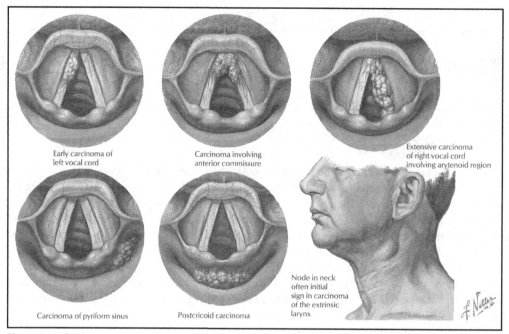

Figure 2-19. Carcinoma at various locations within the larynx. (Netter illustration used with permission of Elsevier, Inc. All rights reserved. www.netterimages.com.)

THE ORAL-MOTOR SYSTEM, LARYNX, AND RESPIRATORY SYSTEM IN RELATIONSHIP WITH CARCINOMA OF THE LARYNX

Now that each major system that is central to speech, chewing, swallowing, and respiration has been outlined, a brief discussion of how carcinoma can compromise the unique interplay of these systems' support of these life-sustaining and communicative functions are discussed briefly. Laryngeal cancer may invade the larynx at any number of sites from one or both vocal folds to surrounding structures (Figure 2-19) and can even spread supraglottically to the oral-motor system and subglottically to the structures of the respiratory system (i.e., trachea). Starting at the level of the glottis, if a tumor invades one or both vocal folds, the ability of the folds to close off and protect the airway may be compromised depending on the size of the cancer and how deep within the vocal fold tissue it is located. In some cases, the cancer may restrict vocal fold movement, leading to a lack of vocal fold closure and the risk of foreign materials leaving the oral-motor system and entering the trachea below the folds instead of being diverted into the esophagus behind the trachea. If LC extends superiorly from the glottis and spreads to structures such as the ventricular folds and epiglottis, these other levels of protection for preventing aspiration of materials into the airway will likely be compromised also.

As can be imagined, a lack of vocal fold closure will further compromise phonation by preventing the vocal folds from adducting together to build up air pressure from the respiratory system and power vocal fold vibration. In addition, the vibratory characteristics of the vocal folds are likely to be compromised with the invasion of tumors, because the vocal folds will become stiffer. As a result, higher levels of subglottic pressure must be generated to set the vocal folds into vibration even if they can be initially moved to midline via the LCA, IA, and TA muscles. In some cases, the tumor invading the larynx is so large that it enters the glottis and prevents the vocal folds from allowing air into the respiratory system. If the cancer extends into the glottis and down into the trachea, respiratory function will be affected even more severely and lead to life-threatening consequences beyond those of the cancer itself. In addition, a large lesion that extends into the trachea may impinge on the esophagus and make the transit of food materials from the lower pharynx into the stomach difficult.

If a tumor from the larynx extends into the oral-motor system, it may not be possible to effectively widen and constrict the pharynx and move the tongue, jaw, velum, and lips freely. If this is the case, improper resonance for speech and reduced intelligibility may result. In addition, manipulation of food and liquids in the oral and pharyngeal cavities may be restricted by tumor invasion, leading to an inability to properly chew food or move it safely into the esophagus for transit into the stomach.

CONCLUSION

The interplay between the structures of the oral-motor system, larynx, and respiratory system are paramount for facilitating life-sustaining and communicative functions. An understanding of each of the structures within each component system and how each system broadly works with the others can provide insight into how the presence of LC may impact the ability of these systems to sustain proper nutrition via chewing and swallowing, airway protection, respiration, and communication via phonation, proper resonance, and articulation.

REFERENCES

Agostini, E., & Mead, J. (1964). Statics of the respiratory system. In W. Fenn & H. Rahn (Eds.), *Handbook of physiology, respiration I* (pp. 387-409). Washington, DC: American Physiological Society.

Belafsky, P. C. (2010). Manual control of the upper esophageal sphincter. *The Laryngoscope, 120,* S1-S16.

Hirano, M. (1974). Morphological structures of the vocal cord as a vibrator and its variations. *Folia Phoniatrica, 26,* 89-94.

Hixon, T. J., Weismer, G., and Hoit, J. D. (2013). *Preclinical speech science. Anatomy, physiology, acoustics, perception* (2nd ed). San Diego, CA: Plural.

Kuna, S. T., Insalaco, G., & Woodson, G. E. (1988). Thyroarytenoid muscle activity during wakefulness and sleep in normal adults. *Journal of Applied Physiology, 65,* 1332-1339.

Noordzij, J. P., & Ossoff, R. H. (2006). Anatomy and physiology of the larynx. *Otolaryngology Clinics of North America, 39,* 1-10.

Rothenberg, M. (1983). An interactive model for the voice source. In D. Bless & J. Abbs (Eds.), *Vocal fold physiology: Contemporary research and clinical issues* (pp. 155-165). San Diego, CA: College-Hill Press.

Shiotani, A., Westra, W. H., & Flint, P. W. (1999). Myosin heavy chain composition in human laryngeal muscles. *The Laryngoscope, 109,* 1521-1524.

Shipp, T. (1975). Vertical laryngeal position during continuous and discrete vocal frequency change. *Journal of Speech and Hearing Research, 18,* 707-718.

Titze, I. R. (1994). *Principles of voice production.* Englewood, Cliffs, NJ: Prentice-Hall.

Wade, O. L., & Gilson, J. C. (1951). The effect of posture on diaphragmatic movements and vital capacity in normal subjects with a note on spirometry as an aid in determining radiological chest volumes. *Thorax, 6,* 103-126.

van den Berg, J. (1958). Myoelastic-aerodynamic theory of voice production. *Journal of Speech and Hearing Research, 1,* 227-244.

Wu, Y. Z., Crumley, R. L., Armstrong, W. B., & Caiozzo, V. J. (2000). New perspectives about human laryngeal muscle: Single-fiber analyses and interspecies comparisons. *Archives of Otolaryngology-Head & Neck Surgery, 126,* 857-864.

Zemlin, W. (1998). *Speech and hearing science: Anatomy and physiology.* Boston, MA: Allyn & Bacon.

SUGGESTED READINGS

Boone, D. R., McFarlane, S. C., Von Berg, S. L., & Zraick, R. L. (2013). *The voice and voice therapy* (9th ed.). New York, NY: Pearson.

McFarland, D. H. (2015). *Netter's atlas of anatomy for speech, swallowing, and hearing* (2nd ed.). St. Louis, MO: Mosby.

Moses, K. P., Banks, J. C., Nava, P. B., & Petersen, D. K. (2013). *Atlas of clinical gross anatomy* (2nd ed.). Philadelphia, PA: Elsevier, Inc.

Newlands, S. D., Calhoun, K. H., Curtin, H. D., Deskin, R.W., Eibling, D. E. Ferguson, B. J., ... Toriumi, D. M. (2006). *Head & Neck Surgery–Otolaryngology* (4th ed.). Philadelphia, PA: Lippincott Williams & Wilkins.

Seikel, J. A., King, D. W., & Drumright, D. G. (2010). *Anatomy & physiology for speech, language, and hearing* (4th ed.). Clifton Park, NY: Delmar-Cengage Learning.

West, J. B. (2012). *Respiratory physiology* (9th ed.). Baltimore, MD: Lippincott Williams & Wilkins.

3

Medical and Surgical Diagnosis and Treatment of Laryngeal Cancer

*Connor W. Hoban, BS; Paul L. Swiecicki, MD; and
Andrew G. Shuman, MD*

INTRODUCTION TO MANAGING LARYNGEAL CANCER

Laryngeal cancer (LC) poses a substantial threat to many facets of a patient's well-being. Because of the intimate relationship between anatomy and physiology in the head and neck, LC can damage structures that play a key role in life-sustaining and quality-of-life–promoting functions. To address the aggressive nature of tumor-related morbidity in patients with LC, it is typically best practice for multidisciplinary health care teams (MDTs) to work with patients to carefully plan and support their treatment. Oncologic considerations and patient preferences must be carefully balanced to ensure that selected therapies are engineered to individually accommodate patients' needs and desired outcomes. Consequently, multiple perspectives, including those of head and neck surgeons, medical oncologists, radiation oncologists, and many other providers, are indispensable for optimal LC management.

INDIVIDUALIZED ASSESSMENT OF LARYNGEAL CANCER

Once the diagnosis of LC is confirmed, further characterization of the disease is necessary for optimal management. Many descriptive aspects of a tumor, including its location, involvement of local structures, and metastatic distribution, collectively assign the cancer to a categorical stage that helps to predict disease behavior and the most appropriate treatment. Appropriate classification of the cancer enables health care teams to make informed decisions and practice personalized medicine.

Friberg, J. C., & Vinney, L. A.
*Laryngeal Cancer: An Interdisciplinary
Resource for Practitioners* (pp. 45-58).
© 2017 Taylor and Francis Group.

Additional considerations are also obligatory for treatment planning. Nearly every cancer diagnosis imparts an arduous physical and emotional demand on the patient. Moreover, these formidable challenges are often exacerbated by the treatment course itself. Therefore, the potential impact of a patient's overall health, functional status, and medical comorbidities on his or her candidacy for various treatments must be considered. Holistic consideration of the tumor stage/biology, anticipated functional outcomes, quality of life, and established patient preferences enable MDTs to formulate the optimal treatment regimens (van Wersch et al., 1997).

Workup After Initial Diagnosis

The initial workup demands a concerted effort to better understand the status of the disease and the patient to predict the tumor's anticipated behavior and response to treatment. Patients typically present with changes in voice, difficulty and/or pain with swallowing, painless neck masses, or any combination of these features (Shah, Patel, & Singh, 2012). An advanced malignancy can impinge on the airway. However, the presentation of LC is immensely variable and location dependent, and the workup needs to be individualized. A thorough physical examination of the head and neck, including assessment of voice and swallowing, in patients with suspected LC is imperative for definitively establishing the diagnosis and disease status (Cummings, Haughey, & Thomas, 2005). This examination is typically augmented with in-office *flexible* or *rigid fiberoptic laryngoscopy* to both map the tumor and exclude secondary primary lesions (Cummings et al., 2005).

Biopsy

Biopsy of either the primary tumor and/or cervical lymph node metastasis is necessary to confirm a suspected diagnosis. Consideration of airway patency and safety, often in conjunction with anesthesiology, is necessary before any procedure/intervention (Chu, Lee, & Chang, 2011). Biopsy of the primary tumor is often performed during *direct laryngoscopy* in the operating room, at which point the tumor is mapped and characterized. However, selected tumors may be amenable to tissue collection and examination with the use of local anesthetic and fiberoptic–guided biopsy in the clinic rather than in the operating room (Naidu, Noordzij, Samim, Jalisi, & Grillone, 2012).

Imaging

Appropriate imaging is paramount to the characterization and staging of LC. In addition to identifying synchronous primary tumors and metastases, imaging studies reveal critical information, including the tumor's physical dimensions, specific anatomical coordinates, and extension of the primary tumor (Hermans, Bogaert, Rijnders, Doornaert, & Baert, 1999). Another key component of imaging is its role in guiding surgical and nonsurgical treatment planning (Nguyen et al., 2013).

Imaging of patients with early-stage LC (those with smaller tumors and no clinical evidence of lymph node metastasis) may be less extensive than that completed for those with later-stage tumors. For example, patients with less advanced tumors may not require cross-sectional imaging or radiologic imaging that uses advanced techniques such as computed tomography (CT) and *magnetic resonance imaging* (MRI) to image axial slices of the body. Patients who do not require cross-sectional imaging typically undergo a chest x-ray, which images the chest in two rather than three dimensions, to exclude lung metastases or other primary tumors (Geurts et al., 2006).

In contrast, CT and MRI scans are often used to characterize LC when locoregional extension is suspected (Kuhn et al., 2014). Both of these modalities can depict the primary tumor burden and its intricate relationship with the surrounding anatomy more accurately than endoscopic and physical examinations alone (Zinreich, 2002), and they provide more detailed images than can traditional x-rays. Specifically, imaging cervical lymph nodes is an essential component of the assessment of many LCs (Lindberg, 1972; Zinreich, 2002), especially because larger and more aggressive primary tumors, and those that involve the supraglottic or subglottic larynx, confer a higher risk of cervical metastases (Welsh, Welsh, & Rizzo, 1989). Available methods for characterizing lymph node involvement include ultrasound, MRI, CT, and *positron emission tomography* (PET) *scans* (Zinreich, 2002). The decision to use a specific imaging modality is often decided in concert with the MDT and is influenced by the individualized nature of the malignancy and treatment planning thereof (Zinreich, 2002).

Evaluation of Health Status

Beyond assessments via biopsy and imaging, careful evaluation of a patient's nutrition, dental health, and ability to speak and swallow can intimately guide the management of individualized disease. Proper nourishment, for instance, is a powerful predictor of positive oncologic outcomes (Kubrak et al., 2010). Moreover, radiotherapy (RT) is well known to inflict late toxicities that should be considered before treatment (Vissink, Burlage, Spijkervet, Jansma, & Coppes, 2003). Likewise, an assessment of swallowing function can elucidate additional functional concerns and enables the MDT to consider compromised deglutition in treatment planning (Chu & Kim, 2008). In addition to functional feeding and swallowing, dental health should also be considered. Impaired dental health leads to increased rates of *osteoradionecrosis* or bone death caused by radiation near the head and neck. Awareness of this possible adverse effect guides practitioners in their delivery of radiation therapy and preventive dental care (Duarte et al., 2014; Katsura et al., 2008). Voice is another clinical factor that provides meaningful insight in the optimal management of LC. Vocal fold mobility and pretreatment function are the best predictors of a patient's postoperative functional and survival outcomes (Gorphe et al., 2015). Thus, if the larynx is greatly impaired before treatment or it is suspected that treatment approaches are likely to result in permanent inability to eat and/or communicate effectively, *laryngeal preservation* treatment may be unwarranted (Gorphe et al., 2015).

Staging of Laryngeal Cancer

Accurately staging LC is critical for planning the optimal management. As mentioned in Chapter 1, the American Joint Committee on Cancer of the American Cancer Society uses the TNM staging system, which provides a common language for guiding treatment plans and estimating prognostic outcomes (Greene, Compton, Fritz, Shah, & Winchester, 2006). Within this categorical staging system, individual stages are selected that best describe the anatomical properties of the primary tumor (T), cervical lymph node involvement (N), and distant metastasis (M). Several of these stages are categorized according to organ-specific standards. For LC, for example, the T stage is influenced by the tumor subsite and extension to specific features of the larynx and nearby structures (Greene et al., 2006). The T, N, and M stages of tumors in a given patient contribute to an overall cancer stage or prognostic group that ranges from I to IV (Greene et al., 2006).

Beyond the TNM staging schema, MDTs maintain an awareness of key aspects of laryngeal physiology and typical progression/presentation of LC. For instance, tumors in the supraglottic and subglottic regions have a higher proclivity for lymphatic (regional) and distant metastatic spread at the time of diagnosis (Welsh et al., 1989). In addition, physicians often regard early-stage primary tumors without clinically evident nodal disease as being unlikely to present with distant metastases (Foote, 2007). This knowledge is important in treatment planning and overall disease management.

Prognostic Considerations in Laryngeal Cancer

The cancer staging system is widely regarded as having pertinent prognostic quality (Dansky Ullmann, Harlan, Shavers, & Stevens, 2012). According to the TNM algorithm, patients with early-stage cancers (I or II) have an average 5-year survival rate of 85%, and those with advanced-stage cancer (III or IV) have closer to a 50% 5-year survival rate (Forastiere et al., 2003; Pointreau et al., 2009). However, the TNM staging system overlooks other criteria that have been shown to be prognostic (Emerick et al., 2013). As a result, several individualized online prognosis calculators are now available to patients with cancer and health practitioners to supplement the TNM system and facilitate predictions regarding LC outcomes (Montero et al., 2014). Outcome calculators often account for recognized prognostic criteria including age, race, sex, comorbidity status, history of smoking and alcohol use, differentiation, histological type, and anatomical subsite. As a result, these calculators can provide improved predictions for overall survival, disease-free survival, functional outcome, and additional measures of clinical significance (Egelmeer et al., 2009).

INDIVIDUALIZED MANAGEMENT OF LARYNGEAL CANCER

After the assignment of a stage for LC, the MDT turns its focus to treatment. Best practices in treatment planning facilitate individualized care, designed to address each patient's physical needs and his or her priorities regarding quality-of-life considerations.

Formulating a Treatment Plan

The balance between oncologic and functional outcomes in patients with LC contributes to the complexity of treatment choices (Pfister et al., 2006). After assessing individual patient factors and associated tumor characteristics, MDTs interact with the patient to consider several important factors:

- Potential voice and swallowing outcomes

- The intensity and length of therapy

- Treatment outcomes based on individualized prognostic factors

In addition, institutional and practical factors often determine the availability of specialized care; these factors include the experience and bias of the practitioner and accessibility of resources, all of which can intimately shape the provision of individualized treatment.

Thoroughly counseling the patient on survival rates and functional outcomes associated with various treatment options is critical for identifying his or her innate preferences (Shuman et al., 2013). Special care should be allocated to assessing the emotional response that patients have toward the prospect of losing their voice and/or living with a tracheostomy, laryngectomy, or feeding tube, all of which can greatly influence post-treatment quality of life (Pfister et al., 2006). Moreover, a patient's financial situation, geographic limitations, and network of social support can be essential in determining the most successful and individualized treatment option. Patients who are eligible for RT, for instance, must have the resources to travel to a facility daily for up to 7 weeks to adhere to the regimen. As a consequence, it is essential to identify patients who might not have access to readily available transport or finances, among other privileges, and recognize that alternative solutions may be required.

The Role of Multidisciplinary Health Care Teams in Treatment Planning

To process this spectrum of information related to treatment decisions, MDTs must meet and collaborate to formulate treatment protocols. MDTs are becoming increasingly prevalent and enable health specialists to align their expertise and offer distinct insights that ultimately tailor treatment plans and target patients' desired outcomes (Fennell, Das, Clauser, Petrelli, & Salner, 2010). MDTs often consider a broad range of factors relating to the tumor, patient, institution, and clinicians to arrive at an individualized option (Foote, 2007). As reviewed in Chapter 1, MDTs, including allied health professionals such as speech-language pathologists, dietitians, respiratory therapists, and social workers, work in concert with physicians on the MDT. In particular, surgeons, medical oncologists, and radiation oncologists provide critical perspectives on the primary treatment approaches for patients with LC. Studies have shown that the broader perspective and holistic considerations promoted by MDTs improve oncologic decision making and optimize clinical outcomes (Burton et al., 2006).

An inevitable aspect of cancer treatment is the reality that treatment may not always be curative in nature. For patients with an advanced-stage cancer, alleviating suffering and bolstering quality of life are regarded as successful outcomes when they decide that they would prefer to embark on a palliative treatment course (Shuman, Yang, Taylor, & Prince, 2011). Because of the value that many patients place on palliation when faced with *head and neck cancer*, the risk of disease persistence and threats to functional outcomes need to be stressed as they relate to their decision to accept or decline certain interventions. When incorporating this communicative transparency into the delivery of care, patients are empowered with the ability to weigh short- and long-term sacrifices against respective therapeutic options and thereby select a strategy that best meets their personal goals for care. Chapter 8 provides additional information related to palliation for patients with LC.

Patients and their families are important members of the MDT. Thus, it is imperative that they be recruited to optimize their own health and wellness, especially given that head and neck cancer imparts a profound challenge to a patient's health status. For example, to facilitate the best possible patient outcomes, tobacco-cessation counseling is obligatory (Decker & Goldstein, 1982; Freedman, Abnet, Leitzmann, Hollenbeck, & Schatzkin, 2007), and nutritional, physical, and emotional wellness is truly paramount to patients' recovery from a tumor and/or treatment effects.

Managing Early-Stage Laryngeal Cancer

Early-stage LC is defined as stage I (T1, N0, M0) or II (T2, N0, M0) disease. Such tumors are typically localized to a specific part of the larynx and have not destroyed vital components of the laryngeal architecture (Compton et al., 2012). As a consequence, early-stage LC is frequently targeted with single-modality treatments (surgery or radiation) that have demonstrated excellent oncologic and functional outcomes. Surgery and radiation are thought to result in similar response and cure rates for patients with early-stage disease (Hinerman et al., 2002; Mendenhall, Amdur, Morris, & Hinerman, 2001); however, few prospective clinical studies have directly compared the treatment outcomes achieved with each modality in patients with stage I or II cancer (Dey et al., 2002). Thus, the choice to pursue radiation versus surgery may be based primarily on specific tumor characteristics and patient and clinician factors (Table 3-1).

Primary considerations include the associated risks of surgery versus those of radiation, posttreatment vocal outcomes, and available modalities for salvage treatment in the event of tumor persistence/recurrence.

Surgical Treatment for Early-Stage Laryngeal Cancer

Surgery for early-stage LC is designed to extirpate the tumor while preserving phonation and swallowing. Conservation (i.e., larynx-preserving) surgery can be performed endoscopically with

TABLE 3-1		
FACTORS THAT INFLUENCE TREATMENT CHOICES IN LARYNGEAL CANCER		
TUMOR CHARACTERISTICS	**PATIENT VARIABLES**	**CLINICIAN VARIABLES**
• Stage • Location • Extension • Pretreatment voice and swallowing function	• Functional status • Comorbidities • Symptom burden • Vocal use patterns • Vocal handicap • Swallowing ability • Preferences and priorities • Social factors, including occupation, support structure, geographic proximity to treatment facilities, and any financial concerns that may be present (Foote, 2007)	• Experience and bias of the treatment team • Availability of and access to necessary equipment and facilities

or without a laser (without a skin incision in the neck and via surgical manipulations to the larynx via endoscopes placed through the mouth or nose) or as open surgery (directly through a skin incision in the neck). Transoral laser resection via endoscopy is common practice for early-stage LC surgery (Sesterhenn, Dünne, & Werner, 2006); however, this approach requires meticulous technique to eradicate tumors and preserve function (Remacle et al., 2010). A patient's candidacy for transoral resection depends on how easily the endoscope can visualize his or her entire tumor site as well as the location of disease (Foote, 2007). More aggressive resections done as a result of more extensive tumors typically engender worse vocal outcomes (Remacle et al., 2007). In certain cases of early-stage LC (typically involving sites other than the glottis), *occult* cervical lymph node involvement (microscopic metastasis that is not visible or palpable) must be considered. For these patients, elective *neck dissection* may be included in the primary treatment plan (Case Study 3-1).

Radiation Treatment for Early-Stage Laryngeal Cancer

As previously noted, external beam radiation is thought to be as effective as surgical approaches in treating early-stage LC. Radiation oncologists devise therapeutic treatment regimens that typically involve daily doses of radiation over a duration that can range from 2 to 7 weeks (Foote, 2007). Fractionation schemas (how radiation dosing is divided over ensuing days and sessions) can vary. In all cases, radiation therapy is designed specifically to address the tumor and associated at-risk areas and to spare healthy tissues. Decisions about radiation dosage, timing, duration, and exposure are made on the basis of individual patient considerations and should be discussed thoroughly with the MDT.

Managing Advanced-Stage Laryngeal Cancer

As many as two-thirds of all patients with head and neck cancer present with advanced disease at the time of diagnosis (Argiris, Karamouzis, Raben, & Ferris, 2008). Advancements in therapeutic techniques and their delivery have facilitated practitioners' effective treatments of advanced

---

CASE STUDY 3-1

PATIENT NAME: FRANCINE

Clinical Status: stage I laryngeal cancer

Francine presented with a 3-month history of hoarseness and was diagnosed with a suspicious mass in her larynx. Direct operative laryngoscopy with biopsy and subsequent radiologic imaging confirmed stage I (T1b, N0, M0) squamous cell carcinoma of her true vocal cords.

Francine was counseled that single-modality treatment with either radiation therapy or endoscopic resection is a reasonable option for her early-stage cancer and that she has an excellent prognosis. The MDT believed that the anatomy of her tumor was such that her predicted voice outcome might be slightly better with radiation therapy. However, Francine is highly motivated to complete treatment quickly and get back to work, and she is less concerned with her voice. She underwent successful surgery and is currently doing very well. After her surgery, Francine is being monitored by members of the MDT for post-surgical assessment and survivorship care.

---

disease, each of which carries a distinct set of risks and benefits (Laccourreye et al., 2012; Yang et al., 2009). Thus, the MDT and all of its members are critical for designing and prioritizing treatments based on their unique consequences and likely effect on disease (Laccourreye et al., 2012; Yang et al., 2009).

Unlike that for early-stage LC, effective management of advanced LC commonly requires multiple therapeutic modalities (Szuecs et al., 2015). Available treatments fit into one of the following two overarching categories based on whether larynx preservation is feasible and/or indicated:

1. Primary total laryngectomy with subsequent RT or chemoradiotherapy is indicated for very advanced local tumors and those that have led to irreversible laryngeal dysfunction.

2. Larynx-preservation protocols for advanced disease include RT, conservation surgery with or without RT or chemoradiotherapy, concurrent chemoradiotherapy, and *induction chemotherapy* followed by RT or chemoradiotherapy (Szuecs et al., 2015).

The advent of effective larynx-preserving protocols is a cornerstone of the management of LC and is attractive to patients when feasible and indicated. Larynx-preservation efforts are often successful in maintaining laryngeal function, but patient selection is paramount (Carrara-de Angelis, Feher, Barros, Nishimoto, & Kowalski, 2003). Larynx-preservation strategies that result in the loss of natural voice (see Chapter 5), respiratory difficulty (see Chapter 4), and/or swallowing dysfunction (see Chapter 6)—with or without tumor control—are likely inferior to total laryngectomy (Szuecs et al., 2015). Various approaches to surgical treatment of LC are described in the following sections.

Conservation Surgery

Conservation surgery involves partial resection of the larynx. These selective laryngectomy procedures remain as a viable option to specifically remove advanced-stage tumors while maintaining native laryngeal function (Forastiere, Weber, & Trotti, 2015). Transoral laryngeal microsurgery is a surgical technique that can be used to resect portions of the larynx in certain advanced tumors (Hinni et al., 2007). Refinements in transoral laryngeal microsurgery and careful patient selection for conservation surgery, along with the provision of *adjuvant therapy* when appropriate, has resulted in low tracheotomy and gastrostomy rates and impressive oncologic outcomes in many patients with advanced disease (Hinni et al., 2007).

Total Laryngectomy

Total laryngectomy continues to be an essential oncologic procedure for advanced LC. The operation involves gross excision of the larynx and varying extents of surrounding tissue and lymphatics (Remacle et al., 2010). Pathologic risk-adjusted adjuvant RT with or without chemotherapy is frequently indicated after laryngectomy and is based on characterization of the tumor's biology and its appearance under the microscope after it has been surgically removed (Remacle et al., 2010). Survival outcomes equal and sometimes exceed those observed with organ-sparing protocols in population data analyses (Hoffman et al., 2006).

Total laryngectomy subjects patients to a dramatic transformation that can intimately infringe on their quality of life (Laccourreye et al., 2012). The absence of a larynx forces patients to breathe through their neck, relinquish their natural voice, and forfeit their sense of smell (Timon & Reilly, 2006). However, many patients can learn to speak, eat, and regain most levels of pretreatment function after surgery. Broaching the subject of total laryngectomy involves a rigorous discussion and demands an extraordinary measure of transparency, counseling, and empathy. This conversation helps to properly align patient preference with MDT insight and thereby helps the MDT strive for an optimum individualized outcome (Shuman, Fins, & Prince, 2012).

Advances in Larynx Preservation

The profound finding that select patients can undergo definitive nonsurgical intervention with laryngeal preservation and without sacrifice in overall survival revolutionized the oncologic approach to advanced-stage LC management. Specifically, the Veterans' Administration Laryngeal Cancer Study Group first provided evidence for this principle when they compared the effectiveness of induction chemotherapy, which consisted of cisplatin and fluorouracil (PF), with adjuvant RT to the standard regimen, total laryngectomy and adjuvant RT (Wolf et al., 1991). Patients in the induction chemotherapy arm were evaluated after two cycles of this first phase of treatment for tumor response (Wolf et al., 1991). Patients whose cancer did not respond to the induction chemotherapy were treated with total laryngectomy followed by adjuvant RT (Wolf et al., 1991). Patients whose cancer responded to the original treatment completed one more course of chemotherapy before undergoing adjuvant RT (Wolf et al., 1991). The Veterans' Administration Laryngeal Cancer Study Group confirmed that almost two of three patients who underwent the larynx-preserving regimen kept their larynx 3 years after treatment, and no difference in 5-year overall survival rates between the two study arms was found (Wolf et al., 1991).

After establishing the feasibility of laryngeal preservation via nonsurgical intervention in patients with advanced disease, many efforts ensued to refine optimal regimens and improve functional outcomes without sacrificing survival rates. The Intergroup Radiation Therapy Oncology Group 91-11 (RTOG 91-11) study was a prospective randomized trial that specifically compared the administration of (1) concurrent chemotherapy (cisplatin) and RT versus (2) induction chemotherapy (cisplatin and fluorouracil) with subsequent radiation versus (3) radiation therapy alone (Forastiere et al., 2003). Concurrent chemoradiotherapy conferred the best laryngeal preservation after 10 years (Forastiere et al., 2013). Longitudinal follow-up studies to the RTOG 91-11 reported similar overall survival rates among the study arms (Forastiere et al., 2013).

The French Group for Head and Neck Oncology Radiotherapy (GORTEC) study was another pioneering randomized clinical trial that aimed to validate the efficacy and utility of multimodality laryngeal preservation protocols by using an induction chemotherapy approach (Pointreau et al., 2009). This study demonstrated that a triplet drug induction that consisted of paclitaxel, cisplatin, and fluorouracil elicited a greater response rate and therefore subjected fewer patients to total laryngectomy than chemotherapy that consisted of paclitaxel and fluorouracil or PF doublet drug induction (Pointreau et al., 2009).

Harnessing targeted therapies likely represents the future of cancer treatment. Cetuximab is a targeted chemotherapy drug that consists of a monoclonal antibody that facilitates endothelial growth factor receptor inhibition and is the only currently available and approved targeted agent for head

---

CASE STUDY 3-2

PATIENT NAME: MELVIN

Clinical Status: stage IVa laryngeal cancer

Melvin presented with a 6-month history of a slowly growing neck mass, *odynophagia*, and weight loss. Clinical examination revealed an ulcerative tumor on his epiglottis and multiple suspicious lymph nodes in his neck. Direct operative laryngoscopy with biopsy and subsequent radiologic imaging confirmed stage IVa (T3, N2b, M0) squamous cell carcinoma of his supraglottic larynx.

Melvin's main treatment goal, other than cure, was to maintain his larynx. He understood the relative tradeoffs between different organ-preservation approaches, and he was keen to ensure that his odds of saving his larynx were high before committing to radiation. He was treated with a chemoselection induction chemotherapy protocol and experienced good initial response to treatment; thus, he started undergoing definitive chemoradiation and had a complete response to therapy. Members of the MDT now provide Melvin with supportive care to promote successful nutrition and communication throughout and after treatment.

---

and neck cancer (Forastiere et al., 2015). However, a recent prospective study tempered enthusiasm for the role of cetuximab in the primary treatment of locoregionally advanced LC when it found that the drug did not provide a significant improvement in survival outcomes (Forastiere et al., 2015; Lefebvre et al., 2013). Its role in adjuvant and other settings is more apparent.

Clinical researchers continue to determine how best to use chemotherapy and RT to maximize oncologic and functional results while limiting *toxicity* and recognizing the inherent tumor biology. The Veterans' Administration Laryngeal Cancer Study Group first described induction chemotherapy as a mechanism for guiding subsequent treatment on the basis of initial response to chemotherapy (Urba et al., 2006). The principle of chemoselection built on this foundation by incorporating one cycle of induction chemotherapy (PF) and consequently evaluating tumor response in more recent prospective studies (Urba et al., 2006; Vainshtein et al., 2013) (Case Study 3-2).

Navigating Treatment Approaches

Induction chemotherapy, concurrent chemoradiation, and surgery with adjuvant therapy offer essentially equivalent oncologic outcomes to patients with advanced LC. However, the decision process to select one of these modalities is highly patient dependent and significantly influenced by individualized tumor parameters, the patient's preoperative health status, the provider's expertise, and the patient's preference. The goal of optimizing functional outcomes persists as a defining factor in these treatment initiatives and often carries substantial weight when considered on a patient-to-patient basis. Collaborations during multidisciplinary conferencing enable health teams to tailor treatment strategies that focus on patient preference, consider medical context, and accommodate individual circumstances (including financial status, social support, and access to transportation) to deliver optimal patient care.

SALVAGE TREATMENT FOR RECURRENT LARYNGEAL CANCER

After suspicion and discovery of recurrent LC, diligent imaging, staging, and multidisciplinary assessment are obligatory and should parallel the initial work-up described earlier in this chapter

(Motamed, Laccourreye, & Bradley, 2006). Any treatment of recurrent LC is considered salvage treatment and, similar to initial treatment, requires consideration of tumor factors, patient factors, and multidisciplinary input. Consideration of previous treatment, the time since initial treatment, tissue integrity, overall health, and the risk of associated complications guide salvage intervention (Crevoisier et al., 1998; Janot et al., 2008).

Prognosis and quality of life are two significant considerations that can affect the relative indications and advantages of salvage treatment modalities. Decisions to pursue salvage modalities will likely exacerbate pre-existing challenges. As a consequence, counseling patients on realistic therapeutic outcomes and taking into account their preferences are of paramount importance (List et al., 1996). Furthermore, it is likely that only a restricted subpopulation of patients will truly benefit from salvage procedures. Identifying these patients is critical for mitigating treatment toxicity among those who are unlikely to experience significant prolongation of life (Crevoisier et al., 1998). Variables to consider include the disease-free interval, functional status, previous treatment, and pretreatment/post-treatment disease stage.

Resectable laryngeal tumors that recur after radiation therapy are best treated via surgery. In many of these cases, *salvage total laryngectomy* is required; however, some patients may be candidates for *salvage partial (conservation) laryngectomy* (Motamed et al., 2006). Management of the cervical lymph nodes in the salvage setting is personalized similarly. *Salvage surgery* often confers the risk of a higher incidence of complications and regularly requires complex reconstructive procedures to promote optimal postoperative function and successful healing (Weber et al., 2003).

Salvage treatment can also be performed using radiation (or reirradiation) with or without chemotherapy (Crevoisier et al., 1998; Janot et al., 2008). Critical considerations include previous radiation exposure, the time since treatment, the effects of previous treatment and current disease on the tissue site, tumor stage before and after treatment, and functional factors such as performance status, symptom burden, and swallowing ability.

LARYNGEAL CANCER SURVIVORSHIP

The optimal provision of survivorship care follows the successful management of cancer and consists of avid surveillance for tumor recurrence, mitigation of treatment effects, and active promotion of wellness. Regular screening for locoregional recurrence, distant metastasis, and second primary tumors is driven by established guidelines. Optimal surveillance protocols include consideration of individualized patient criteria and are typically de-escalated over time as the risk of recurrence decreases (Foote, 2007).

Despite offering increased efficacy, modern therapies subject patients to substantial toxicities that can impede quality of life and threaten the preservation of many vital facets of human functionality (Turner, 2015). This reality necessitates longitudinal evaluation of physical health, mental wellness, and quality of life (List et al., 1996). Patients often develop an extensive host of late complications including dry mouth, dysphagia, dental disease, and hypothyroidism, among many other concerns (Foote, 2007; So et al., 2012; Vissink et al., 2003). Similar to many patients with cancer, LC survivors also face chronic pain, fatigue, and depression (Carlson, Waller, Groff, Giese-Davis, & Bultz, 2013). Mindful anticipation and mitigation of these adverse effects serves to enhance quality of life and consequently improves patient outcomes. Persistent tobacco use is a potent predictor of decreased control of disease and survival. Thus, tobacco-cessation counseling is critical (Browman et al., 1993).

INCURABLE LARYNGEAL CANCER

Advanced unresectable locoregional or distant metastatic LC, either at initial diagnosis or recurrence, is considered incurable and is a source of significant morbidity and death. Current cancer-directed treatment protocols consider palliative surgery (metastasectomy of distant lesions) and/or radiation for control of tumor burden and symptoms in select cases (Young, Diakos, Khalid-Raja, & Mehanna, 2015). More frequently, a palliative regimen of systemic chemotherapy is used to decrease tumor burden and slow progression of the disease.

First-line chemotherapy in patients with an acceptable performance status consists of a pharmaceutical triplet (a platinum agent and fluorouracil plus cetuximab) that has been shown to provide the best overall survival rate among patients with incurable disease to date (Colevas, 2006; Gibson et al., 2005; Vermorken et al., 2008). However, selecting a specific therapeutic regimen, including the number and type of agents, remains dependent on patient preferences, comorbidities, and performance status. Immunotherapeutic agents are in development and preclinical studies have demonstrated their successful recruitment of patients' inherent immune system to target cancer (Chow et al., 2014).

All palliative regimens can engender formidable toxicities and thereby reinforce the need for careful consideration of patient status and palliative intent when considering end-of-life cancer management (Sacco & Cohen, 2015). Elaborate discussions between the MDT and the patient should concern functional status, expected outcomes, associated toxicities, and desired palliation to address the complexities of incurable cancer care delivery (Sacco & Cohen, 2015).

CONCLUSION

Laryngeal cancer targets a delicate organ that empowers patients with critical components of human functionality. The inherent threat to viable functional and survival outcomes thereby poses a profound challenge to patients and health care providers combating this disease. Although surgery, radiation therapy, and chemotherapy are all potential treatment options, deciding on a cohesive treatment plan is often complicated. Multidisciplinary collaborations between professionals should welcome patients to contribute to their own management choices. Such partnerships promote considerations of oncologic, clinician, and patient factors that are invaluable for the design of individualized interventions. Establishing synergy between practitioners and patients enables teams to effectively navigate the intricate nature of LC management and pursue surgical and nonsurgical modalities that reflect patient preferences and optimize desired outcomes.

REFERENCES

Argiris, A., Karamouzis, M. V., Raben, D., & Ferris, R. L. (2008). Head and neck cancer. *The Lancet, 371*, 1695–1709.

Browman, G. P., Wong, G., Hodson, I., Sathya, J., Russell, R., McAlpine, L., ... Levine, M. N. (1993). Influence of cigarette smoking on the efficacy of radiation therapy in head and neck cancer. *New England Journal of Medicine, 328*, 159–163.

Burton, S., Brown, G., Daniels, I. R., Norman, A. R., Mason, B., Cunningham, D., & Royal Marsden Hospital Colorectal Cancer Network. (2006). MRI directed multidisciplinary team preoperative treatment strategy: The way to eliminate positive circumferential margins? *British Journal of Cancer, 94*, 351–357.

Carlson, L. E., Waller, A., Groff, S. L., Giese-Davis, J., & Bultz, B. D. (2013). What goes up does not always come down: Patterns of distress, physical and psychosocial morbidity in people with cancer over a one-year period. *Psycho-Oncology, 22*, 168–176.

Carrara-de Angelis, E., Feher, O., Barros, A., Nishimoto, I., & Kowalski, L. (2003). Voice and swallowing in patients enrolled in a larynx preservation trial. *Archives of Otolaryngology–Head & Neck Surgery, 129*, 733–738.

Chow, L. Q. M., Eaton, K. D., Baik, C., Goulart, B., Morishima, C., Disis, M. L., … Martins, R. G. (2014). Phase 1b trial of TLR8 agonist VTX-2337 in combination with cetuximab in patients with recurrent or metastatic squamous cell carcinomas of the head and neck (SCCHN). *International Journal of Radiation Oncology, Biology, Physics, 88,* 503–504.

Chu, E. A., & Kim, Y. J. (2008). Laryngeal cancer: Diagnosis and preoperative work-up. *Otolaryngologic Clinics of North America, 41,* 673–695.

Chu, P. Y., Lee, T. L., & Chang, S. Y. (2011). Impact and management of airway obstruction in patients with squamous cell carcinoma of the larynx. *Head & Neck, 33,* 98–102.

Colevas, A. D. (2006). Chemotherapy options for patients with metastatic or recurrent squamous cell carcinoma of the head and neck. *Journal of Clinical Oncology, 24,* 2644–2652.

Compton, C. C., Byrd, D. R., Garcia-Aguilar, J., Kurtzman, S. H., Olawaiye, A., & Washington, M. K. (2012). Larynx. In C. C. Compton, D. R. Byrd, J. Garcia-Aguilar, S. H. Kurtzman, A. Olawaiye, & M. K. Washington (Eds.), *AJCC cancer staging atlas* (pp. 79–90). New York, NY: Springer.

Crevoisier, R. D., Bourhis, J., Domenge, C., Wibault, P., Koscielny, S., Lusinchi, A., … Eschwege, F. (1998). Full-dose reirradiation for unresectable head and neck carcinoma: Experience at the Gustave-Roussy Institute in a series of 169 patients. *Journal of Clinical Oncology, 16,* 3556–3562.

Cummings, C. W., Haughey, B. H., & Thomas, J. R. (2005). *Cummings otolaryngology: Head & neck surgery* (4th Ed. Review). Philadelphia, PA: Elsevier Mosby.

Dansky Ullmann, C., Harlan, L. C., Shavers, V. L., & Stevens, J. L. (2012). A population-based study of therapy and survival for patients with head and neck cancer treated in the community: Therapy and survival in H&N cancer. *Cancer, 118,* 4452–4461.

Decker, J., & Goldstein, J. C. (1982). Risk factors in head and neck cancer. *New England Journal of Medicine, 306,* 1151–1155.

Dey, P., Arnold, D., Wight, R., MacKenzie, K., Kelly, C., & Wilson, J. (2002). Radiotherapy versus open surgery versus endolaryngeal surgery (with or without laser) for early laryngeal squamous cell cancer. *The Cochrane Database of Systematic Reviews,* (2), CD002027.

Duarte, V. M., Liu, Y. F., Rafizadeh, S., Tajima, T., Nabili, V., & Wang, M. B. (2014). Comparison of dental health of patients with head and neck cancer receiving IMRT vs conventional radiation. *Otolaryngology–Head and Neck Surgery, 150,* 81–86.

Egelmeer, A. G. T. M., de Jong, J. M., Dehing, C., Boersma, L., Kremer, B., & Lambin, P. (2009). 8509 Development of a nomogram for prediction of survival and local control in larynx carcinoma treated with radiotherapy alone: A cohort study based on 994 patients. *European Journal of Cancer Supplements, 7,* 473.

Emerick, K. S., Leavitt, E. R., Michaelson, J. S., Diephuis, B., Clark, J. R., & Deschler, D. G. (2013). Initial clinical findings of a mathematical model to predict survival of head and neck cancer. *Otolaryngology–Head and Neck Surgery, 149,* 572–578.

Fennell, M. L., Das, I. P., Clauser, S., Petrelli, N., & Salner, A. (2010). The organization of multidisciplinary care teams: Modeling internal and external influences on cancer care quality. *JNCI Monographs, 2010,* 72–80.

Foote, R. L. (2007). Radiotherapy alone for early-stage squamous cell carcinoma of the larynx and hypopharynx. *International Journal of Radiation Oncology, Biology, Physics, 69,* S31–S36.

Forastiere, A. A., Goepfert, H., Maor, M., Pajak, T. F., Weber, R., Morrison, W., … Cooper, J. (2003). Concurrent chemotherapy and radiotherapy for organ preservation in advanced laryngeal cancer. *New England Journal of Medicine, 349,* 2091–2098.

Forastiere, A. A., Weber, R. S., & Trotti, A. (2015). Organ preservation for advanced larynx cancer: Issues and outcomes. *Journal of Clinical Oncology, 33,* 3262–3268.

Forastiere, A. A., Zhang, Q., Weber, R. S., Maor, M. H., Goepfert, H., Pajak, T. F., … Cooper, J. S. (2013). Long-term results of RTOG 91–11: A comparison of three nonsurgical treatment strategies to preserve the larynx in patients with locally advanced larynx cancer. *Journal of Clinical Oncology, 31,* 845–852.

Freedman, N. D., Abnet, C. C., Leitzmann, M. F., Hollenbeck, A. R., & Schatzkin, A. (2007). Prospective investigation of the cigarette smoking–head and neck cancer association by sex. *Cancer, 110,* 1593–1601.

Geurts, T. W., Ackerstaff, A. H., Van Zandwijk, N., Hart, A. a. M., Hilgers, F. J. M., & Balm, A. J. M. (2006). The psychological impact of annual chest x-ray follow-up in head and neck cancer. *Acta Oto-Laryngologica, 126,* 1315–1320.

Gibson, M. K., Li, Y., Murphy, B., Hussain, M. H. A., DeConti, R. C., Ensley, J., & Forastiere, A. A. (2005). Randomized phase III evaluation of cisplatin plus fluorouracil versus cisplatin plus paclitaxel in advanced head and neck cancer (E1395): An intergroup trial of the Eastern Cooperative Oncology Group. *Journal of Clinical Oncology, 23,* 3562–3567.

Gorphe, P., Blanchard, P., Breuskin, I., Temam, S., Tao, Y., & Janot, F. (2015). Vocal fold mobility as the main prognostic factor of treatment outcomes and survival in stage II squamous cell carcinomas of the glottic larynx. *Journal of Laryngology & Otology, 129,* 903–909.

Greene, F. L., Compton, C. C., Fritz, A. G., Shah, J. P., & Winchester, D. P. (2006). *AJCC cancer staging atlas.* New York, NY: Springer.

Hermans, R., Van den Bogaert, W., Rijnders, A., Doornaert, P., Baert, A.L., (1999). Predicting the local outcome of glottic squamous cell carcinoma after definitive radiation therapy: value of computed tomography-determined tumour parameters. *Radiotherapy Oncology, 150*(1), 39–46.

Hinerman, R. W., Mendenhall, W. M., Amdur, R. J., Stringer, S. P., Villaret, D. B., & Robbins, K. T. (2002). Carcinoma of the supraglottic larynx: Treatment results with radiotherapy alone or with planned neck dissection. *Head & Neck, 24,* 456–467.

Hinni, M. L., Salassa, J. R., Grant, D. G., Pearson, B. W., Hayden, R. E., Martin, A., … Steiner, W. (2007). Transoral laser microsurgery for advanced laryngeal cancer. *Archives of Otolaryngology–Head & Neck Surgery, 133,* 1198–1204.

Hoffman, H. T., Porter, K., Karnell, L. H., Cooper, J. S., Weber, R. S., Langer, C. J., … Robinson, R. A. (2006). Laryngeal cancer in the United States: Changes in demographics, patterns of care, and survival. *Laryngoscope, 116,* 1–13.

Janot, F., de Raucourt, D., Benhamou, E., Ferron, C., Dolivet, G., Bensadoun, R.-J., … Bourhis, J. (2008). Randomized trial of postoperative reirradiation combined with chemotherapy after salvage surgery compared with salvage surgery alone in head and neck carcinoma. *Journal of Clinical Oncology, 26,* 5518–5523.

Katsura, K., Sasai, K., Sato, K., Saito, M., Hoshina, H., & Hayashi, T. (2008). Relationship between oral health status and development of osteoradionecrosis of the mandible: A retrospective longitudinal study. *Oral Surgery, Oral Medicine, Oral Pathology, Oral Radiology, and Endodontics, 105,* 731–738.

Kubrak, C., Olson, K., Jha, N., Jensen, L., McCargar, L., Seikaly, H., … Baracos, V. E. (2010). Nutrition impact symptoms: Key determinants of reduced dietary intake, weight loss, and reduced functional capacity of patients with head and neck cancer before treatment. *Head & Neck, 32,* 290–300.

Kuhn, F. P., Hüllner, M., Mader, C. E., Kastrinidis, N., Huber, G. F., von Schulthess, G. K., … Veit-Haibach, P. (2014). Contrast-enhanced PET/MR imaging versus contrast-enhanced PET/CT in head and neck cancer: How much MR information is needed? *Journal of Nuclear Medicine, 55,* 551–558.

Laccourreye, O., Malinvaud, D., Holsinger, F. C., Consoli, S., Ménard, M., & Bonfils, P. (2012). Trade-off between survival and laryngeal preservation in advanced laryngeal cancer: The otorhinolaryngology patient's perspective. *Annals of Otology, Rhinology & Laryngology, 121,* 570–575.

Lefebvre, J. L., Pointreau, Y., Rolland, F., Alfonsi, M., Baudoux, A., Sire, C., … Bardet, E. (2013). Induction chemotherapy followed by either chemoradiotherapy or bioradiotherapy for larynx preservation: The TREMPLIN randomized phase II study. *Journal of Clinical Oncology, 31,* 853–859.

Lindberg, R. (1972). Distribution of cervical lymph node metastases from squamous cell carcinoma of the upper respiratory and digestive tracts. *Cancer, 29,* 1446–1449.

List, M. A., Ritter-Sterr, C. A., Baker, T. M., Colangelo, L. A., Matz, G., Pauloski, B. R., & Logemann, J. A. (1996). Longitudinal assessment of quality of life in laryngeal cancer patients. *Head & Neck, 18,* 1–10.

Mendenhall, W. M., Amdur, R. J., Morris, C. G., & Hinerman, R. W. (2001). T1-T2No squamous cell carcinoma of the glottic larynx treated with radiation therapy. *Journal of Clinical Oncology, 19,* 4029–4036.

Montero, P. H., Yu, C., Palmer, F. L., Patel, P. D., Ganly, I., Shah, J. P., … Patel, S. G. (2014). Nomograms for preoperative prediction of prognosis in patients with oral cavity squamous cell carcinoma. *Cancer, 120,* 214–221.

Motamed, M., Laccourreye, O., & Bradley, P. J. (2006). Salvage conservation laryngeal surgery after irradiation failure for early laryngeal cancer. *Laryngoscope, 116,* 451–455.

Naidu, H., Noordzij, J. P., Samim, A., Jalisi, S., & Grillone, G. A. (2012). Comparison of efficacy, safety, and cost-effectiveness of in-office cup forcep biopsies versus operating room biopsies for laryngopharyngeal tumors. *Journal of Voice, 26,* 604–606.

Nguyen, N. P., Kratz, S., Lemanski, C., Vock, J., Vinh-Hung, V., Gorobets, O., … Ampil, F. (2013). Image-guided radiotherapy for locally advanced head and neck cancer. *Radiation Oncology, 3,* 172.

Pfister, D. G., Laurie, S. A., Weinstein, G. S., Mendenhall, W. M., Adelstein, D. J., Ang, K. K., … Wolf, G. T. (2006). American society of clinical oncology clinical practice guideline for the use of larynx-preservation strategies in the treatment of laryngeal cancer. *Journal of Clinical Oncology, 24,* 3693–3704.

Pointreau, Y., Garaud, P., Chapet, S., Sire, C., Tuchais, C., Tortochaux, J., … Calais, G. (2009). Randomized trial of induction chemotherapy with cisplatin and 5-fluorouracil with or without docetaxel for larynx preservation. *Journal of the National Cancer Institute, 101,* 498–506.

Remacle, M., Eckel, H. E., Chevalier, D., Quer, M., Perretti, G., & Werner, J. (Eds.). (2010). *Surgery of larynx and trachea.* Berlin: Springer.

Remacle, M., Haverbeke, C. V., Eckel, H., Bradley, P., Chevalier, D., Djukic, V., … Werner, J. (2007). Proposal for revision of the European Laryngological Society classification of endoscopic cordectomies. *European Archives of Oto-Rhino-Laryngology, 264,* 499–504.

Sacco, A. G., & Cohen, E. E. (2015). Current treatment options for recurrent or metastatic head and neck squamous cell carcinoma. *Journal of Clinical Oncology, 33,* 3305–3313.

Sesterhenn, A. M., Dünne, A. A., & Werner, J. A. (2006). Complications after CO_2 laser surgery of laryngeal cancer in the elderly. *Acta Oto-Laryngologica, 126,* 530–535.

Shah, J. P., Patel, S. G., & Singh, B. (2012). *Head and neck surgery and oncology.* Philadelphia, PA: Elsevier Health Sciences.

Shuman, A. G., Fins, J. J., & Prince, M. E. (2012). Improving end-of-life care for head and neck cancer patients. *Expert Review of Anticancer Therapy, 12,* 335–343.

Shuman, A. G., McCabe, M. S., Fins, J. J., Kraus, D. H., Shah, J. P., & Patel, S. G. (2013). Clinical ethics consultation in patients with head and neck cancer. *Head & Neck, 35,* 1647–1651.

Shuman, A. G., Yang, Y., Taylor, J. M. G., & Prince, M. E. (2011). End-of-life care among head and neck cancer patients. *Otolaryngology–Head and Neck Surgery, 144,* 733–739.

So, W. K. W., Chan, R. J., Chan, D. N. S., Hughes, B. G. M., Chair, S. Y., Choi, K. C., & Chan, C. W. H. (2012). Quality-of-life among head and neck cancer survivors at one year after treatment—A systematic review. *European Journal of Cancer, 48,* 2391–2408.

Szuecs, M., Kuhnt, T., Punke, C., Witt, G., Klautke, G., Kramp, B., & Hildebrandt, G. (2015). Subjective voice quality, communicative ability and swallowing after definitive radio(chemo)therapy, laryngectomy plus radio(chemo) therapy, or organ conservation surgery plus radio(chemo)therapy for laryngeal and hypopharyngeal cancer. *Journal of Radiation Research, 56,* 159–168.

Timon, C., & Reilly, K. (2006). Head and neck mucosal squamous cell carcinoma: Results of palliative management. *Journal of Laryngology & Otology, 120,* 389–392.

Turner, J. (2015). Engaging patients in survivorship care planning after completion of treatment for head and neck cancer. *Cancer Forum, 39,* 101.

Urba, S., Wolf, G., Eisbruch, A., Worden, F., Lee, J., Bradford, C., ... Taylor, J. (2006). Single-cycle induction chemotherapy selects patients with advanced laryngeal cancer for combined chemoradiation: A new treatment paradigm. *Journal of Clinical Oncology, 24,* 593–598.

Vainshtein, J. M., Wu, V. F., Spector, M. E., Bradford, C. R., Wolf, G. T., & Worden, F. P. (2013). Chemoselection: A paradigm for optimization of organ preservation in locally advanced larynx cancer. *Expert Review of Anticancer Therapy, 13,* 1053–1064.

van Wersch, A., de Boer, M.F., van der Does, E., de Jong, P., Knegt, P., Meeuwis, C.A., Stringer, P., Pruyn, J.F. (1997). Continuity of information in cancer care: evaluation of a logbook. *Patient Education and Counseling, 31*(3), 223–36.

Vermorken, J. B., Mesia, R., Rivera, F., Remenar, E., Kawecki, A., Rottey, S., ... Hitt, R. (2008). Platinum-based chemotherapy plus cetuximab in head and neck cancer. *New England Journal of Medicine, 359,* 1116–1127.

Vissink, A., Burlage, F. R., Spijkervet, F. K. L., Jansma, J., & Coppes, R. P. (2003). Prevention and treatment of the consequences of head and neck radiotherapy. *Critical Reviews in Oral Biology & Medicine, 14,* 213–225.

Weber, R. S., Berkey, B. A., Forastiere, A., Cooper, J., Maor, M., Goepfert, H., ... Ensley, J. (2003). Outcome of salvage total laryngectomy following organ preservation therapy: The radiation therapy oncology group trial 91–11. *Archives of Otolaryngology–Head & Neck Surgery, 129,* 44–49.

Welsh, L. W., Welsh, J. J. & Rizzo T. A. (1989). Internal anatomy of the larynx and the spread of cancer. *Annals of Otology, Rhinology and Laryngology, 98,* 228–234.

Wolf, G. T., Hong, W. K., Fisher, S. G., Urba, S., Endicott, J. W., Close, L., ... Fye, C. (1991). Induction chemotherapy plus radiation compared with surgery plus radiation in patients with advanced laryngeal cancer. *New England Journal of Medicine, 324,* 1685–1690.

Yang, E. S., Murphy, B. M., Chung, C. H., Netterville, J. L., Burkey, B. B., Gilbert, J., ... Cmelak, A. J. (2009). Evolution of clinical trials in head and neck cancer. *Critical Reviews in Oncology/Hematology, 71,* 29–42.

Young, E. R., Diakos, E., Khalid-Raja, M., & Mehanna, H. (2015). Resection of subsequent pulmonary metastases from treated head and neck squamous cell carcinoma: Systematic review and meta-analysis. *Clinical Otolaryngology, 40,* 208–218.

Zinreich, S. J. (2002). Imaging in laryngeal cancer: Computed tomography, magnetic resonance imaging, positron emission tomography. *Otolaryngologic Clinics of North America, 35,* 971–991.

4

Airway and Respiratory Challenges in Laryngeal Cancer

Lisa Crujido, MS, CCC-SLP

Airway management is a critical consideration in the treatment of advanced laryngeal cancer (LC). Because of the proximity of the larynx to major respiratory structures, laryngeal tumors or reactions to cancer treatments may compromise breathing. As such, securing and maintaining a patent airway may become a primary concern for the patient and for the head and neck surgeon treating him or her.

This chapter describes two surgical procedures, tracheostomy and partial/total laryngectomy, that are frequently performed during treatment for LC. The impact of these procedures on the respiratory system is explained, and information related to the care and management of artificial airways is also offered.

THE RESPIRATORY PROCESS

Recall that Chapter 2 provided extensive information about the process of respiration and the anatomy and physiology needed for breathing and airway patency. Beyond understanding how respiration works, it is important to understand contributions of the nasal cavity to normal respiration.

The Nasal Cavity

The functions of the human nose are quite diverse and include providing an airway, a filtration and humidification system (i.e., a thermoregulator that warms air during nasal inspiration), a resonating chamber for speech production, and a receptor for olfaction. Approximately

Friberg, J. C., & Vinney, L. A.
Laryngeal Cancer: An Interdisciplinary Resource for Practitioners (pp. 59-72).
© 2017 Taylor and Francis Group.

10,000 to 20,000 liters of air move daily through the nasal cavity to the lungs during normal respiration (Wang, Li, Yan, Li, & Shi, 2015). The anatomical design of the interior nose (i.e., nasal septum and turbinates), coupled with the shape of the external nose, changes the aerodynamics of airflow from a laminar flow (air flowing in parallel streams) at the nasal vestibule to a highly turbulent flow (unsteady air with fluctuating velocity flowing in many directions) at the inferior turbinate (Wang, Lee, & Gordon, 2012). This change in airflow facilitates the mucosal contact that is needed for filtration and humidification of inspired air. During nasal breathing, ambient air, with a temperature of 22°C and relative humidity of 40%, is warmed and humidified by the upper airway to reach a temperature of up to 32°C and a relative humidity of up to 99% at the level of the trachea (Bien, Okla, van As-Brooks, & Ackerstaff, 2010). The ability of the nose to thermoregulate the air passing through it creates an optimal condition for *mucociliary lavage* or the clearance of foreign materials via cilia and mucous in the nose, trachea, and bronchi.

Olfaction

The olfactory system represents one of the oldest sensory modalities in the phylogenetic history of mammals. Olfaction occurs when odorant molecules within inspired air make contact with the epithelium of the olfactory bulb, located high in the nasal cavity. There are multiple fibers that project to the olfactory cortex via the olfactory tract, which contains both subcortical and cortical projections and enables smell to be registered (Hadley, Orlandi, & Fong, 2004). During eating, retronasal olfaction occurs in the oropharynx. Instead of the direct nasal inhalation of odorant particles during typical olfaction, the acts of chewing and swallowing allow a small amount of these particles to pass through the nasopharynx to the nose so that specific flavors can be identified (Hadley et al., 2004). Because a patient with a laryngectomy or tracheotomy (discussed later) breathes through the neck, he or she will be unable to engage in olfaction during quiet breathing but may report awareness of odors when eating as a result of retronasal olfaction.

Upper and Lower Airway Structures and Functions

The anatomy of the normal respiratory system can be organized into the upper and lower respiratory tracts. The upper respiratory tract consists of the structures superior to the larynx, and the lower respiratory tract includes structures inferior to the larynx. It is important to note that the larynx acts as the connection between the upper and lower airways, and the vocal folds abduct and adduct to modulate airflow throughout the respiratory system. Thus, the larynx serves an important function for respiration, and any dysfunction or disease at the level of the larynx can disrupt respiration and affect a person's ability to breathe. Figure 4-1 illustrates the relationship between the upper and lower airways.

RESPIRATION DYSFUNCTION

When a patient is diagnosed with LC, a tumor has grown in the vicinity of the vocal folds, which can result in inefficient or abnormal vocal fold function depending on the size and location of the tumor. Even if the vocal folds initially function normally, tumor growth or swelling and other tissue changes (i.e., *fibrosis*) from curative treatments (e.g., radiation) can eventually affect laryngeal function and have subsequent effects on respiration. When such a situation occurs, patients may need to undergo a surgical procedure called a tracheotomy to establish a safe and patent airway.

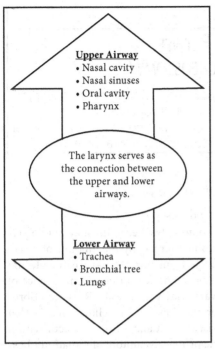

Figure 4-1. Upper and lower airway physiology.

Tracheotomy

A tracheotomy is an incision into the trachea via the neck. This incision is maintained as a hole called a *stoma* (sometimes called a *tracheostoma*), which allows for breathing to occur by way of the neck. A tracheotomy can be performed for airway management at the following junctures:

- Before any surgical treatment of the tumor (i.e., laryngectomy)
- Before or in conjunction with medical treatments for LC (e.g., chemoradiation)
- At the same time as a laryngectomy
- Preventively for cases in which chronic dysphagia is likely and/or maintenance or pulmonary hygiene will be required

When a tracheotomy is performed, the respiratory function of the oral/nasal tracts is bypassed through the placement of a *tracheostomy tube* (Box 4-1). As a result, the tracheostomy tube enables patients to inhale and exhale and exchange oxygen and carbon dioxide through the tracheostomy rather than their mouth or nose.

Because respiration is managed via the neck after tracheotomy, rather than the upper respiratory system, patients who undergo a tracheotomy are sometimes referred to as *neck breathers*. Despite airflow being directed through the neck after a tracheotomy, there can be residual airflow through the nose and mouth after surgery. The amount of residual air depends on the type of tracheostomy tube used and the degree of obstruction that is superior to the tube itself. Factors that influence the amount of this obstruction include the following:

- Width of the patient's glottal opening during respiration (i.e., the amount of vocal fold abduction)
- Amount of space occupied by the mass in the hypopharynx or supraglottic, glottic, or subglottic airway
- Degree of supraglottic, glottic or subglottic edema
- Amount of laryngeal or tracheal stenosis or injury (if any)

Box 4-1

WHAT IS THE DIFFERENCE BETWEEN A TRACHEOTOMY AND A TRACHEOSTOMY?

Although these terms sound similar, they are not synonymous. Dikeman and Kazandjian (2003) describe a tracheotomy as the "surgical creation of an opening in the trachea" (p. 56) to allow for an alternative path for respiration and a tracheostomy as an artificial airway maintained with a tracheostomy tube placed in the stoma after a tracheotomy.

- Whether airway reconstruction occurred after tracheal or laryngeal surgery
- The onset of fibrosis or internal/external *lymphedema* and its severity

In patients with intact upper airway structures and functions, a tracheostomy may not be permanent. The need for a permanent tracheostomy is determined largely by the amount of resection that is required for tumor management, adverse effects from nonsurgical treatment, and the ultimate integrity and function of the larynx. Fibrosis of the neck is often a consequence of radiation therapy with or without chemotherapy and can vary widely in severity. Radiation fibrosis, defined as a dysregulated, excessive, and autocrine production of extracellular matrix that leads to progressive stiffening of the connective tissue (Krisciunas et al., 2015), can occur within months to years after the completion of treatment. Thus, the primary symptom of radiation fibrosis, as a consequence of radiation to the larynx, is reduced range of motion in the neck and loss of laryngeal mobility. Vertical range of motion, which is critical for swallowing and phonation and for lateromedial range of motion, which is necessary for vocal fold abduction and adduction, may be impaired. This loss of lateromedial movement of the vocal folds reduces the glottal opening, which is essential for airway patency. The need for a tracheotomy also depends on how well the patient tolerates his or her compromised airway; however, in most cases, a glottal opening of 3 mm or less requires tracheotomy to prevent or decrease symptoms of dyspnea and enable adequate oxygen intake.

Tracheostomy Tubes

Tracheostomy tubes can be metal or plastic and vary in size. There are three basic components to a tracheostomy tube:

1. An *outer cannula* (main body of the tracheostomy tube) that functions to keep the artificial airway in place and can be secured to the neck externally
2. An *inner cannula* that fits inside the outer cannula via a locking mechanism
3. An *obturator*, which fits inside the outer cannula to provide a smooth rounded surface for guiding insertion of the outer and inner cannulas; the obturator is removed once the cannulas are in place (Figure 4-2 provides an image of each of these components)

Tracheostomy tubes are kept in place using cloth ties or Velcro straps that are attached to the faceplate of the outer cannula and secured around the neck. The outer cannula may contain a *cuff* or small balloon (see Figure 4-2) that when inflated, a complete seal is achieved between the tracheostomy tube and tracheal wall. This closed system is necessary for mechanical ventilation and the seal further reduces the risk of aspiration. A cuffed tracheostomy is typically used when a patient requires mechanical ventilation or is at risk for frank aspiration. Many patients who require long-term use of tracheostomy tubes without ventilation do very well with metal cuffless tubes. Figure 4-3 provides a visual of a tracheostomy tube positioned in a person with intact laryngeal anatomy.

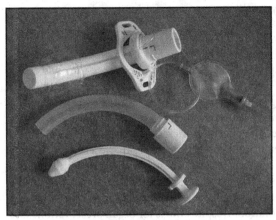

Figure 4-2. Components of a tracheostomy tube, including outer cannula (top) and inflatable cuff (top right), inner cannula (center), and obturator (bottom). (Reprinted with permission from Peter Klaus at https://commons.wikimedia.org/wiki/File:Tracheostomy_tube.jpg#file.)

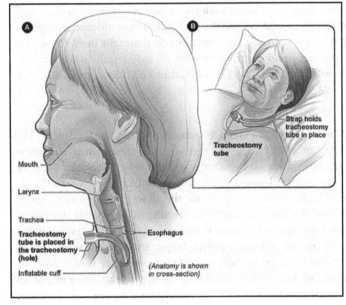

Figure 4-3. Position of tracheostomy tube internally and externally in a patient with intact laryngeal anatomy. (Reprinted with permission from National Heart Lung and Blood Institute [NIH] [public domain], via Wikimedia Commons at https://upload.wikimedia.org/wikipedia/commons/e/ed/Tracheostomy_NIH.jpg.)

Tracheostomy Care

The tracheostomy tube can be cleaned by removing the inner cannula and using a brush, warm water, and hydrogen peroxide as either a flush or a soak. In addition, daily use of a saline flush instilled into the tracheal opening for pulmonary lavage and cleaning of the inner cannula is recommended. A *speaking valve* (e.g., the Passy-Muir or Montgomery) enables voice production and facilitates a more natural swallow while improving secretion management and oxygenation. A cloth or foam stoma cover is useful for filtration; however, many patients with a tracheostomy find it unnecessary, especially those who wear a speaking valve or a tracheostomy *decannulation button*. It is important to remember that most tracheostomized patients will demonstrate multi-modality air exchange (tracheostomy, nasal, and oral breathing). Patients receive extensive training in tracheostomy care before leaving the hospital.

Laryngeal Cancer Treatment and Airway Patency

Chapter 3 describes medical and surgical treatment options, including radiation, chemotherapy, and partial/total laryngectomy, for patients with LC. Outside of airway issues that can arise from the simple presence of a tumor in the larynx, these treatments for LC can also affect airway patency.

Medical Treatment for Laryngeal Cancer

Many patients with LC desire nonsurgical approaches to treatment to preserve the anatomical function of the larynx for communication and respiration. Thus, they pursue chemotherapy and/or radiation to shrink or eliminate their laryngeal tumor. In fact, with advances in chemoradiation regimens, organ preservation has been a sought-after treatment for more advanced (i.e., stages T3 and T4) LCs. In the past three decades, there has been an increase in the use of nonsurgical treatments for cancer of the larynx (Hoffman et al., 2006). Yet, despite organ preservation, airway management considerations remain a central concern because these patients often still require an artificial airway as a result of treatment effects. In a study of 109 patients with a tumor of the base of the tongue, larynx, or hypopharynx, Langerman, Patel, Cohen, and Blair (2012) examined airway management in patients before chemoradiation. Despite efforts for organ preservation, 43% of these patients required *debulking* (surgical removal of part of a tumor when complete excision is not possible) or tracheotomy. Patients with a stage T4 supraglottic tumor or cancer with deep invasion into adjacent structures are often not candidates for debulking and may ultimately require a tracheotomy during chemoradiation or partial/total laryngectomy to maintain their respiratory function. Overall, any patient who pursues medical treatments for LC may require a tracheotomy as a result of treatment effects (e.g., significant edema after radiation) or tumor growth if treatments are unsuccessful (Case Study 4-1).

Surgical Treatment for Laryngeal Cancer

Some patients with advanced LC must undergo a laryngectomy as part of their treatment. This procedure requires the removal of part or all of the larynx to maximize treatment effectiveness. Surgical removal of part or all of the larynx via laryngectomy has obvious implications for respiration. Patients facing total laryngectomy will lose a vital component of respiration as the larynx, specifically the vocal folds, serve as the protective valve for the airway. A surgically-created, permanent airway is established during the reconstruction that results in a complete disconnect of the upper and lower airways. For patients with a tumor that originated from the epiglottis, aryepiglottic folds, false vocal folds, or true vocal folds, a partial laryngectomy may be performed. This technique may minimize morbidity while potentially maintaining the three functions of the larynx (i.e., airway protection, respiration, and phonation). Thus, because the anatomy important for respiration is left intact, it is possible that the patient who undergoes a supraglottic laryngectomy may not require a tracheotomy.

Surgeons commonly perform one of three different types of partial laryngectomy to treat LC:

1. *Supraglottic laryngectomy*: In this surgery, the structures above the level of the vocal folds are resected. This resection includes the false vocal folds and aryepiglottic folds and may be extended to include a single arytenoid, the epiglottis and base of the tongue, and/or the superior, medial, or anterior wall of one or both pyriform sinuses. Thus, because the anatomy important for respiration is left intact, it is possible that the patient who undergoes a supraglottic laryngectomy may not require a tracheotomy.

2. *Hemilaryngectomy (vertical partial laryngectomy)*: In hemilaryngectomy, the thyroid cartilage is divided at midline, and the resection includes one-half of the thyroid cartilage and the corresponding true and false vocal folds and ventricle. Because half of the larynx is removed in a hemilaryngectomy, a tracheotomy may be necessary to overcome the loss of respiratory structure and function.

3. *Near-total laryngectomy*: A near-total laryngectomy is a voice-preserving technique and an option for advanced-stage cancers of the larynx and hypopharynx. In this surgery, portions of the larynx not affected by tumors are spared and often used to reconstruct the larynx. It is a less common approach because of the complexity of the surgery, the limited number of

---

CASE STUDY 4-1

PATIENT NAME: MRS. D. C., A 65-YEAR-OLD WOMAN

Clinical Status: 2 months after diagnosis, 2 weeks into chemoradiation therapy for stage T4 subglottic LC

Comorbidities

- Moderate dysphagia, self-regulating amount and texture of foods to ensure safe, although effortful, swallowing

- Hypertension and gastroesophageal reflux disease, both of which are well controlled via pharmacological means

Initial Assessment Findings

Mrs. D. C. and her doctors determined that because of the location (subglottic, with growth into the cervical spine) and size (4 cm) of her laryngeal tumor, she was not a candidate for safe surgical excision of the cancer. Rather, her immediate treatment goal was to shrink the tumor via chemoradiation and plan for possible partial/total laryngectomy if and when it became safe to do so. At the time of diagnosis, Mrs. D. C. was exhibiting signs of dysphagia because of the size of her tumor; however, her airway, although compromised by the presence of a large laryngeal tumor, was functional for respiration and phonation.

After approximately 2 weeks of chemoradiation therapy, Mrs. D. C. was exhibiting many of the common adverse effects of treatment (i.e., localized swelling, skin irritation, and fatigue). Mrs. D. C.'s family noted that her vocal intensity was diminishing, but they attributed it to her treatment. Shortly thereafter, Mrs. D. C.'s family noted that her mental status seemed altered, it was hard for her to breathe deeply, and at times she seemed to be wheezing. In response to these troubling symptoms, Mrs. D. C. was taken immediately to the hospital. Her otolaryngologist assessed Mrs. D. C. by using a nasoendoscope and found that her trachea was blocked almost completely by her laryngeal tumor (which had grown rather than shrunk during chemoradiation therapy) and swelling associated with her treatment. She was rushed to the operating room for an emergency tracheotomy to create a functional airway for breathing.

Mrs. D. C. stayed in the hospital for several days after the tracheotomy and worked with respiratory therapists, nurses, and speech-language pathologists (SLPs) to learn about secretion management, tracheostomy care, and alternative forms of communication. Because her tumor had grown during treatment, she also worked with her doctors to determine her possible next steps for treatment.

---

surgeons trained in the technique, and the advancement of voice restoration with total laryngectomy. The necessity for a tracheotomy in patients with near-total laryngectomy is dictated entirely by the location of their laryngeal tumor and the physiology that remains after resection.

Although partial laryngectomy is an organ-preservation surgery, it is often only an option for those with early glottic cancer (stage T1 or T2 tumors) or noninvasive disease of the supraglottic structures. The following morbidities related to respiratory function are often associated with partial laryngectomy:

- *Glottic* or *subglottic stenosis*, scarring, or webbing, which results in airway compromise and the need for frequent *tissue resection* and permanent tracheotomy

- Vocal changes caused by poor respiratory drive
- Wound-healing challenges and infection in the larynx that compromise the passage of airflow into the trachea

See Chapters 5 and 6 for additional information on the role of the SLP in managing the impact of these symptoms on communication and swallowing, respectively, in patients with LC.

PULMONARY HYGIENE

An understanding of the relationship of the upper and lower respiratory tract is important for providing the neck-breathing patient with instruction in pulmonary hygiene after a tracheotomy and/or partial/total laryngectomy. The loss of humidification to airflow through the nose can result in reduced clearance of inspired impurities, thickening and crusting of oral/nasal mucus, irritation of the tracheobronchial tree, and overproduction of mucosal secretions (Icuspit, Yarlagadda, Garg, Johnson, & Deschler, 2014). Patients have reported frequent and effortful coughing, excessive sputum production, a dry "tickling" cough, and dyspnea. These symptoms affect both tracheostomized and laryngectomized patients; however, because total laryngectomy patients' sole method of air exchange is via the stoma, *heat- and moisture-exchange systems* (HMEs) often become a necessity.

Heat and Moisture Exchangers

A tracheostoma HME is a system that is recommended for all total *laryngectomees* and is used to aid pulmonary health, patient comfort, and hygiene. Specifically, an HME filters the stoma to humidify the air that moves through it. It is worn over the stoma and consists of a housing and a *foam filter cassette*. The housing can be an external adhesive housing that is disposable or a reusable *lary button* or tube that is placed in the stoma and secured with tracheostomy ties or clips. The foam filter cassettes snap in the housing and are removed before coughing. The cassettes require daily replacement. The benefits of an HME are numerous, and there is a multitude of resources available for patients and families to better understand HME systems. Figure 4-4 provides a visual of an HME in a patient who underwent laryngectomy and *tracheoesophageal puncture* and has a *voice prosthesis*.

In a multicenter study, Ackerstaff et al. (2003) assessed the effects and benefits of HMEs and reported the following findings:

- Reduction in adverse pulmonary symptoms, including less mucus production and easy expectoration of secretions
- Improved sleep as a result of fewer pulmonary problems
- Improved intelligibility via *tracheoesophageal speech* in those with tracheoesophageal puncture (see Chapter 5 for additional information on this topic) because of a decrease in wet and gurgly voice quality
- Overall improvement in postoperative quality of life

MANAGEMENT OF ARTIFICIAL AIRWAYS

Patients with an artificial airway require different supports and medical supplies at different junctures after tracheotomy, particularly immediately after surgery, after their return to home, and in planning return to normal-life roles and responsibilities within the community.

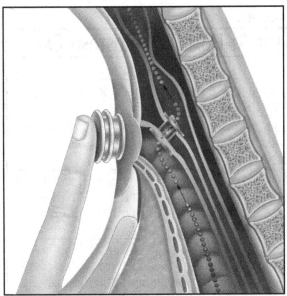

Figure 4-4. An HME placed atop stoma in patient with tracheoesophageal puncture and voice prosthesis. (Reprinted with permission from Laryngectomy 2010 [own work] [CC BY-SA 3.0 (http://creativecommons.org/licenses/by-sa/3.0)], via Wikimedia Commons at https://upload.wiki-media.org/wikipedia/commons/b/be/Heat_and_Moisture_Exchanger.jpg.)

Acute Care Settings

Humidification is critical for pulmonary health and paramount to healing in the days immediately after a tracheotomy or laryngectomy. In most acute care settings, patients spend the first day or two after surgery in an intensive care or intermediate care unit before being transferred to a medical-surgical unit for the remainder of their hospital stay. This unit may contain rooms or a subunit specific to otolaryngology and be staffed with nurses and therapists with extensive experience in managing patients after laryngeal surgery.

Immediately after surgery, patients are fitted with a *tracheostomy mask*, or mist collar that is attached to a nebulizer containing sterile water and an air compressor. The mask is positioned over the stoma to humidify the air breathed in through the neck and may be used intermittently throughout the day or when sleeping at night. During the hospitalization, patients may be fitted with an HME system for long-term humidification of the air that is inspired, especially during daytime activities. Best practice indicates that pulmonary health and healing are facilitated by the use of an HME system in the early stages of recovery. In many cancer centers in the United States, these HME systems are initiated while patients are in an acute care setting with support provided by nursing staff, SLPs, and respiratory therapists, as appropriate. Specifically, instruction in stomal cleaning, pulmonary toileting with *saline bullets*, and the use of humidification is offered to patients and their families:

- The SLP will instruct the patient on the purpose and care of his or her HME system and provide support in any voice prosthesis management and the use of lary tubes and straps.

- Other medical needs, such as wound care, tube-feeding instruction, and stomal protection supplies (shower shields and stoma covers), are addressed by nursing.

- A respiratory therapist may instruct patients in pulmonary suctioning and the use of a tracheostomy mask coupled with an external humidified air system, if needed.

Going Home

Before discharge, a social services representative will arrange for home health services and the delivery of durable medical equipment. The transition to home is eased by support from caregivers

TABLE 4-1	
NECESSARY MEDICAL SUPPLIES FOR AT-HOME TRACHEOSTOMY CARE	
MEDICAL SUPPLY	**PURPOSE**
Suctioning catheters	Suction secretions in and around the tracheostomy tube in the days/weeks after tracheotomy
Alternative communication supports	Supplies such as an *electrolarynx*, a tablet computer, or pen/paper can provide patients with reliable forms of communication after tracheotomy
Heat- and moisture-exchange system	Device that fits over the tracheostomy tube opening and moistens the air that enters the stoma to prevent dryness, thins secretions, and promotes adequate filtering of impurities; often used during daily activity
Humidification system (with or without tracheostomy mask)	Moistens the air that enters the stoma to prevent dryness, thins secretions, and promotes adequate filtering of impurities; often used while sleeping or before a heat- and moisture-exchange system is placed
Laryngectomy tubes	Used immediately after laryngectomy to maintain the opening of the stoma site and prevent stenosis
Tracheostomy straps	Attached to the face plate of a tracheostomy tube's outer cannula to secure it to the neck
Portable suction machine	Machine used to clear secretions from the stoma and inner cannula
Prosthesis-cleaning brush	Provides temporary control of leakage through a current voice prosthesis before it can be changed
Saline bullets	Small capsules of sterile saline that can be used on thickened secretions or dried mucous and provide temporary moisture to the airway in patients with a laryngectomy or tracheotomy
Shower shield	Protective cover that prevents water from entering the stoma during showering and the potential risk of aspiration
Stoma covers	Lightweight, breathable protective cover for the stoma that acts as a filter to keep environmental debris (e.g., dust) from entering the tracheostomy when outside the home and to prevent the expulsion of mucus or secretions through the stoma during sneezing or coughing
Tube-feeding supplies	Facilitate nonoral nutrition for patients who are unable to safely or easily take in food or maintain adequate nutrition by mouth

and medical personnel who will provide ample education and resources to make patients and their families feel comfortable in caring for an artificial airway in the home environment. That said, it may take a neck-breather several months to a full year to adjust to the "new normal," which includes new daily routines and the use of products to support individual needs. Equipment that was needed at home during the early days of surgical recovery will no longer be used; however, there are medical supplies that will be needed throughout the lifetime of the neck-breathing patient. Table 4-1 provides a list of necessary supplies and their purpose for patients who are caring for an artificial airway.

Returning to Community Roles

Planning for functioning outside the home is also important, because these patients will return to previous activities (e.g., work, volunteering, and travel). Thus, they may find it beneficial to assemble supplies for a travel care kit that gives them quick access to stomal care products when they are away from home. The following is a list of supplies that may be helpful to include in a travel care kit for neck-breathing patients:

- HME supplies (e.g., housings, filters, wipes)
- Cleaning supplies for tracheostomy tube components (e.g., brush, saline, cotton swabs)
- Saline bullets (small containers of saline solution for cleaning the stoma site or clearing it of secretions)
- Small flashlight and mirror for visualizing the stoma, tracheoesophageal puncture, or voice prosthesis
- Small pack of tissue or gauze pads for cleaning the area in and around the stoma, tracheo-esophageal puncture, or voice prosthesis
- Extra stomal covers
- Tweezers for delicately removing any crusting or impurities in and around the stoma, tracheo-esophageal puncture, or voice prosthesis

CONCLUSION

For patients with LC, a compromised airway can emerge as a concern at any juncture, from diagnosis through treatment to end-of-life care. Thus, patients should be monitored closely and regularly to ensure continued airway patency and optimal respiratory function. Consider the case of Mr. J. D. (Case Study 4-2) as an example of how airway challenges may affect a patient during and even after treatments for LC.

CASE STUDY 4-2

PATIENT NAME: MR. J. D., AN 82-YEAR-OLD MAN

Clinical Status: 5 years after total laryngectomy for stage T4 squamous cell carcinoma of the larynx; recent secondary tracheoesophageal puncture.

Comorbidities

- Chronic obstructive pulmonary disease; treatments included 2 to 3 liters/minute of supplemental oxygen via tracheostomy mask, bronchodilator inhaler, and daily small-volume nebulizer treatments
- Hypertension, which was well-controlled with medication
- Gastroesophageal reflux disease, which was well-controlled with medication

(continued)

CASE STUDY 4-2 (CONTINUED)

- Mild dysphagia, for which he compensated for by keeping his foods moist and alternating solids and liquids during meals; his weight was stable, and he had been pneumonia free

- *Xerostomia,* for which he frequently chewed gum but did not routinely use over-the-counter products for oropharyngeal hydration

Initial Assessment Findings

Mr. J. D. is an 82-year-old man who is married and lives with his wife in rural southwestern Arizona. He is an avid outdoorsman who loves to travel in his recreational vehicle and participate in horseshoe competitions during travels with his wife. Since his total laryngectomy, his primary method of communication was mostly *esophageal speech* with the occasional use of an electrolarynx. His esophageal speech production was strained with reduced loudness, which made it difficult to be heard in open areas (outdoors) and in large indoor venues. The electrolarynx was cumbersome because it was always getting tangled in his oxygen tubing or getting in the way of him throwing a horseshoe. He was hopeful that having a tracheoesophageal puncture for placement of a voice prosthesis would improve his quality of life. A postsurgical assessment was performed by the SLP, and the following concerns were identified:

- Inconsistent use of stomal covers; the patient admitted that there were times at which he would forget to wear stomal protection, thinking that his tracheostomy mask was providing adequate coverage.

- Loose placement of the tracheostomy mask, with oxygen being delivered as much as 10 to 12 cm from his stoma

- Strained and effortful esophageal speech

- Poor systemic and topical oropharyngeal hydration

- Frequent wet, productive cough with clear to mildly cloudy mucus

- Frequent dry, nonproductive cough

Mr. J. D. was independent in his basic stomal care and had adjusted to changes in his swallowing. He scored high on a quality-of-life scale and looked forward to times spent with his family and friends, travel, and social events. He had a good understanding of the basics (e.g., he is a neck breather who requires oxygen delivery at the stoma, use of a shower shield, and daily pulmonary lavage). He knew the importance of stomal protection for avoiding aspiration; however, his awareness of the purpose of a cover for filtration and humidification was poor.

Instruction on tracheoesophageal voice production was provided, and he was soon able to achieve self-occlusion and a fluent, audible voice. It was evident that Mr. J. D. would have success with his new mode of communication. The SLP's primary concern was his poor pulmonary health.

Because of the asymmetry of his stoma, it was decided that an external housing would provide a better air-tight seal than a lary tube or button. An oval-shaped adhesive housing was chosen, and Mr. J. D. was shown how to place it properly. A foam filter cassette designed for additional humidification was chosen, and the patient was instructed how to place and remove the cassette from the housing.

(continued)

CASE STUDY 4-2 (CONTINUED)

He was asked to wear a heat- and moisture-exchange system around the clock. As long as the adhesive housing maintained a complete seal with no air leak, he was not required to change it daily. The foam filter cassette was to be changed and disposed of after 24 hours of use. Mr. J. D. was shown how to depress the foam filter with his index finger to achieve tracheoesophageal voice.

Recommendations and Goals

- Always wear the HME (24 hours/day, 7 days/week).
- Continue use of supplemental oxygen as prescribed by his pulmonologist, with a cassette in place.
- Remove the foam filter cassette during pulmonary treatments (both bronchodilator inhaler and small-volume nebulizer).
- Increase water intake.
- Add stomal protection (i.e., cloth stoma cover when in a dusty or windy environment).
- Follow-up with the SLP in 1 month.

Mr. J. D. was cautioned that he would likely experience an increase in mucus production for the first few weeks but then the secretions should diminish. If his pulse-oximeter readings fell below the thresholds set by his pulmonologist or if he felt increasing shortness of breath, he was instructed to try an alternative cassette that would allow for greater airflow. If that failed to improve his respiratory effort and increase his oxygen saturation level, he was to discontinue use of the HME system.

One-Month Follow-Up

- 100% compliance with daily wearing of the HME
- Alternated between extra-moisture and high-airflow cassettes
- 50% reduction in the need for small-volume nebulizer treatments
- Pulse-oximeter readings were within threshold values
- Increased mucus production for the first 2 weeks, followed by a dramatic decline
- 75% less coughing

Mr. J. D. continued to require supplemental oxygen; however, the times that he required 3 liters of oxygen were less frequent. His quality of life improved greatly due to decreased coughing and mucus production and an improved level of energy. With his chronic pulmonary disease, the use of an HME was vital for promoting his pulmonary health. Over time, continued use of the HME system may reduce his symptoms further. Now when Mr. J. D. shows up for his horseshoe-pitching competitions, he has an HME in place with his signature bandana for extra protection and good looks.

REFERENCES

Ackerstaff, A. H., Fuller, D., Irvin, M., MacCracken, E., Gaziano, J., & Stachowiak, L. (2003). Multicenter study assessing effects of heat and moisture exchanger use on respiratory symptoms and voice quality in laryngectomized individuals. *Otolaryngology–Head and Neck Surgery, 129,* 705–712.

Bien, S., Okla, S., van As-Brooks, C. J., & Ackerstaff, A. H. (2010). The effect of a heat and moisture exchanger (Provox_HME) on pulmonary protection after total laryngectomy: A randomized controlled study. *European Archives of Otorhinolaryngology, 267,* 429–435.

Dikeman, K. J., & Kazandjian, M. S. (2003). *Communication and swallowing management of tracheostomized and ventilator-dependent adults* (2nd ed.). New York, NY: Delmar Learning.

Hadley, K., Orlandi, R. R., & Fong, K. (2004). Basic anatomy and physiology of olfaction and taste. *Otolaryngologic Clinics of North America, 37,* 1115–1126.

Hoffman, H. T., Porter, K., Karnell, L. H., Cooper, J. S., Weber, R. S., Langer, C. J., ... Robinson, R. A. (2006). Laryngeal cancer in the United States: Changes in demographics, patterns of care, and survival. *The Laryngoscope, S114,* 1–13.

Icuspit, P., Yarlagadda, B., Garg, S., Johnson, T., & Deschler, D. (2014). Heat and moisture exchange devices for patients undergoing total laryngectomy. *ORL–Head and Neck Nursing, 32,* 20–23.

Krisciunas, G. P., Platt, M., Trojanowska, M., Grillone, G. A., Haines, M. A., & Langmore, S. E. (2015). A novel in vivo protocol for molecular study of radiation-induced fibrosis in head and neck cancer patients. *Annals of Otolaryngology, Rhinology, and Laryngology, 125,* 228–234.

Langerman, A., Patel, R., Cohen, E., & Blair, E. (2012). Airway management before chemoradiation for advanced head and neck cancer. *Head & Neck, 34,* 254–259.

Wang, D. Y., Lee, H. P., & Gordon, B. R. (2012). Impacts of fluid dynamics simulation in study of nasal airflow physiology and pathophysiology in realistic human three-dimensional nose models. *Clinical and Experimental Otorhinolaryngology, 5,* 181–187.

Wang, D., Li, Y., Yan, Y., Li, C., & Shi, L. (2015). Upper airway stem cells: Understanding the nose and role for future cell therapy. *Current Allergy & Asthma Reports, 15,* 490.

5

Communication Challenges in Laryngeal Cancer

Philip C. Doyle, PhD, CCC-SLP

IMPACTS OF LARYNGEAL CANCER ON VOICE AND COMMUNICATION

Regardless of anatomical site, a diagnosis of cancer has immediate and long-term implications for both the person with the disease and members of his or her family. As is the case with any serious illness or disease, verbal communication offers a critical means of expressing a range of emotions and one's needs and desires. Verbal communication also serves to provide a direct link between those with a serious health issue and those who can provide the greatest level of support, including not only family members and loved ones but also the range of health care professionals who are charged with their care in the immediate and extended periods after a cancer diagnosis. In the case of cancer of the larynx, and most particularly when the entire larynx needs to be surgically removed, the immediate loss of the normal voice becomes an even greater concern. The loss of one's larynx as a result of cancer via a radical surgical treatment, termed a total laryngectomy, will completely and permanently eliminate the normal mechanism of voice production (Doyle, 1994) and disrupt speech production for communication purposes. As stated by Gotay and Moore (1992), "head and neck cancer strikes at the most basic of human functions—the abilities to communicate, eat, and interact socially" (p. 5).

Given how rapidly medical treatment protocols are initiated in the case of any cancer diagnosis, one's ability to communicate effectively becomes of even greater importance. This is certainly true in the pretreatment and treatment-planning periods, but it also extends into the early and later phases of treatment and over the entire period of posttreatment rehabilitation. Hence, those who undergo total laryngectomy will need to learn and refine alternative methods of verbal communication for the remainder of their lives. When speech is disrupted or lost, social interactions are threatened, coping and adjustment may be challenged, and one's well-being and quality of life are

Friberg, J. C., & Vinney, L. A.
Laryngeal Cancer: An Interdisciplinary Resource for Practitioners (pp. 73-89).
© 2017 Taylor and Francis Group.

Box 5-1
Several excellent resources on conservation laryngectomy can be found in publications by Doyle (1994), Silver, Beitler, Shaha, Rinaldo, and Ferlito (2009), and Timmermans, de Gooijer, Hamming-Vrieze, Hilgers, and van den Brekel (2014).

directly influenced (Blood, Luther, & Stemple, 1992; Hassan & Weymuller, 1993; Karnell, Funk, & Hoffman, 2000).

The type of treatment that is undertaken when a laryngeal cancer (LC) is diagnosed is guided by the size and location of the tumor and an array of other medical factors that determine the staging of the disease. A cancer that is small and well defined and presents without any sign of spread holds the potential for less radical treatment in comparison to larger lesions that cross anatomic boundaries or have spread into the lymphatic system of the neck (Doyle, 1994; Robertson, Yeo, Sabey, Young, & MacKenzie, 2013). Although this chapter focuses on advanced disease that necessitates a total laryngectomy, the reader should be aware that early, smaller, more focal, and less advanced lesions may be treated through the use of radiation therapy (RT) alone or via surgical techniques that are termed conservation surgical procedures (Box 5-1). In partial laryngectomy procedures, less tissue is removed in an effort to retain some degree of a laryngeal voice and/or normal swallowing (Forastiere et al., 2003; Hanna et al., 2004; Hillman, Walsh, Wolf, Fisher, & Hong, 1998).

It also must be pointed out that multiple modalities of treatment, either alone or in combination with one another, may be pursued depending on each person's unique circumstances. Treatment modalities include surgery, RT, and chemoradiation therapy, again depending on the staging of disease specific to the potential for regional or distal spread of the malignancy (Mendenhall et al., 2002). It is equally important to note that in some instances of early lesions, treatment may prove to be unsuccessful; therefore, additional approaches to treatment may be pursued when there is a recurrence of disease. In such circumstances, a secondary surgical treatment termed salvage laryngectomy will be required (Finizia, Hammerlid, Westin, & Lindström, 1998; Robertson et al., 2013). For example, RT that ultimately fails and results in recurrence of the cancer necessitates surgical intervention. As a consequence, the array of potential treatment modalities and the decision for their use derives from multiple factors and considerations. However, for situations in which additional treatment is required because of recurrence, new challenges in the context of posttreatment communication options may emerge with increasing frequency (e.g., salvage laryngectomy after a failed course of RT or chemoradiation treatment may result in an increased potential for complications such as a tissue tear or fistula).

On the basis of the identified considerations, the primary objective of this chapter is to outline the options for verbal communication in the context of total laryngectomy. These postlaryngectomy rehabilitation options are collectively termed alaryngeal voice and speech methods (Box 5-2).

Alaryngeal speech refers to any means of verbal communication that relies on a new nonlaryngeal voice, a source that replaces the signal that was previously provided by the larynx. Accordingly, this chapter includes a description of the basic mechanism of how each of the most commonly used alaryngeal voice and speech methods is achieved and distinguished from one another at multiple levels. In addition, each of these postlaryngectomy verbal communication methods is defined by how the resultant speech is distinctly different from that of the normal speaker. A brief summary of the relative advantages and disadvantages of each method is provided. Despite the obvious limitations that are observed with all postlaryngectomy alaryngeal speech options, this chapter also introduces the reader to information that will permit a fair and balanced consideration of all options available to those who undergo total laryngectomy (Berry, 1978; Doyle, 1994).

BOX 5-2

For the purposes of this chapter, the terms *voice* and *speech* are used independently and collectively. However, it is important to acknowledge that in the strictest definitional form, *voice* refers to the generation of a fundamental sound source, whereas *speech* refers to the modification of the voice source into the distinct sounds of any given language for speech communication purposes.

OVERVIEW OF ALARYNGEAL VOICE AND SPEECH

In the following sections, descriptions of the three most commonly used alaryngeal communication options are presented. However, this is not an exhaustive outline of all possible postlaryngectomy options. Therefore, the following discussion centers on postlaryngectomy verbal communication, that which is generated by the person rather than via methods that employ *augmentative/alternative communication* devices through computer-based options (e.g., text-to-speech generators, synthesized voice). In outlining the multiple options that exist for the rehabilitation of voice and speech in those who undergo total laryngectomy, it should be noted that all of these methods will fall considerably short of the auditory-perceptual characteristics that define the normal human voice (Doyle & Eadie, 2005; Eadie & Doyle, 2005a, 2005b; Eadie, Day, Sawin, Lamvik, & Doyle, 2012).

Postlaryngectomy voice and speech involve alterations of pitch, loudness, and overall voice quality. Such alterations are clearly identifiable to the listener (Bennett & Weinberg, 1973; Doyle & Eadie, 2005; Robbins, Fisher, Blom, & Singer, 1984; Shipp, 1967; Williams & Watson, 1985). Intelligibility may also vary dramatically (Holley, Lerman, & Randolph, 1983; McCroskey & Mulligan, 1963; Weiss & Basili, 1985), with subsequent challenges in the effectiveness of communication and the inherent potential for frustration for both the speaker and the listener (Bjordal, Freng, Thorvik, & Kaasa, 1995; Clements, Rassekh, Seikaly, Hokanson, & Calhoun, 1997; Doyle, 1994). Listeners may be uncomfortable interacting with speakers who use *alaryngeal communication*, which then may negatively affect these speakers' social roles and identities. For example, women who rely on alaryngeal communication methods after total laryngectomy may experience compromised gender identity because of their lowered pitch, the increased noise in the speech they produce, and/or their mechanical voice quality (Brown & Doyle, 1999; Cox & Doyle, 2014; Eadie, Doyle, Hansen, & Beaudin, 2008; Graham & Palmer, 2002; Searl & Small, 2002; Trudeau & Qi, 1990). Thus, there is potential for social stigma as a result of both physical changes to the individual who has undergone laryngectomy and the auditory characteristics of his or her new voice (Cox, Theurer, Spaulding, & Doyle, 2015; Doyle, 1994). However, as already stated, although no alaryngeal method is a perfect replacement for the normal human voice, alaryngeal voice/speech can provide a very good and highly functional mode of verbal communication (Salmon, 2005). These alaryngeal options afford patients the opportunity to resume as full a life as possible after laryngectomy.

Those who have undergone total laryngectomy must be provided fair and balanced information specific to each alaryngeal communication method. With a greater understanding of each of these methods, it is hoped that those who must rely on such approaches after laryngectomy will achieve the most successful verbal communication possible. Accordingly, a brief description of normal anatomy and voice production and the changes that occur as a result of laryngectomy are provided first.

STRUCTURAL AND FUNCTIONAL CHANGES AFTER LARYNGECTOMY

A full understanding of postlaryngectomy communication options initially requires that one understand some of the basic anatomical changes that occur as part of laryngectomy. Knowledge of these changes may facilitate a more thorough understanding of each of the postlaryngectomy communication options that are discussed in later sections of this chapter.

In its normal state, the larynx is positioned at the top of the trachea (airway or windpipe), and its primary biological purpose is to provide airway protection (e.g., preventing aspiration or choking). After a total laryngectomy is performed, the entire laryngeal structure, composed of cartilages and muscles, is dissected from the top of the trachea at the midline of the neck. Recall from Chapter 2 that the larynx normally serves at the transitional anatomical structure between the trachea and lungs and those structures that form the upper airway, including the throat and oral cavity above the larynx. In a normal system, the supraglottis (or vocal tract) is the region above the vocal folds, which includes the upper airway to the lips. Accordingly, this region also includes the throat or pharynx and the oral and nasal cavities, which serve as resonance chambers. The vocal tract provides a very important reference point for normal voice and speech production and for all alaryngeal methods of speech communication. Beginning with this normal point of reference, we can now consider more fully what changes occur as a result of laryngectomy and how these changes influence voice and speech production after total laryngectomy.

When the larynx is surgically removed, the top of the trachea is disconnected from the upper portions of the vocal tract (i.e., the pharynx, oral, and nasal cavities). Thus, once the larynx is removed, the trachea must be brought forward to the anterior midline of the neck, where it is sutured into place just above the sternum (breastbone) in what would normally be referred to as the hollow of the neck. This reconfiguration of the airway results in the creation of what is termed a tracheostoma. The tracheostoma forms the patient's new airway, one that is fully open, visible, and unprotected unless it is covered.

Because the postlaryngectomy airway formed by the newly created tracheostoma is open, significant care must be taken to protect the airway and lungs from any external threat (e.g., dust, water). It is also necessary to mention that the tracheostoma forms the point of breathing, for both inspiration and expiration. Because of this fundamental change, the person who undergoes a total laryngectomy will become a neck breather for the remainder of his or her life. Thus, those who have undergone laryngectomy must be taught to actively protect their airway when involved in daily activities such as bathing. For example, if the laryngectomee leaves the tracheostoma unprotected while showering or swimming, water may enter the lungs through the tracheostoma and result in subsequent aspiration or drowning (Box 5-3).

Adjustments must also be made for other common daily activities. For example, the laryngectomee must be taught to actively cover his or her tracheostoma when coughing, or mucous may be propelled out of the tracheostoma. Consider this coughing example in the context of a communication interaction between one or more individuals and the added concerns it places on what previously was a relatively simple act. In an effort to not only protect the airway but also avoid an unpleasant situation in the presence of others, it is always recommended that the laryngectomee use some type of covering for the stoma. This covering may be a simple bib or a more elaborate commercially available heat- and moisture-exchange stoma device (Hilgers & Ackerstaff, 2005).

The tracheostoma in those who have undergone laryngectomy is a permanent change; this anatomical opening in the neck will never be closed, and respiration will always occur through this direct access to the lungs. In contrast to a tracheotomy, which most frequently results in a temporary change to a person's airway, it is important to note that in the case of laryngectomy, the tracheostoma is permanent. In addition, as a consequence of laryngectomy, the individual's breathing will remain independent of upper airway anatomy and its relationship to the pharynx,

Box 5-3

Despite wide acceptance and encouragement for the use of first-person language specific to clinical populations (i.e., *person who stutters* rather than *stutterer*), the term *laryngectomee* has long been the preferred term used by those who have undergone a total laryngectomy. Hence, this term appears where appropriate throughout this chapter.

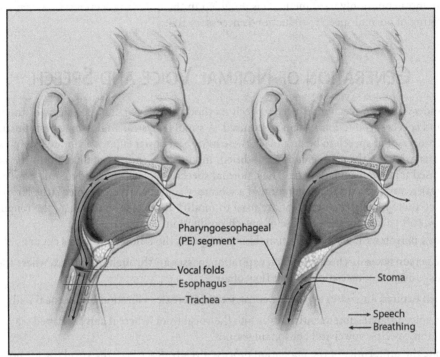

Figure 5-1. Prelaryngectomy (left) and postlaryngectomy (right) alterations in anatomy and the respective relationships between the airway and upper regions of the vocal tract. Directional arrows represent changes in breathing for speech purposes. (Illustration drawn by and reprinted with permission from Dr. Jenna Rebelo, McMaster University, Hamilton, Ontario, Canada.)

oral, and nasal cavities. In the present context, this complete postsurgical separation between previously integrated regions of the lungs, larynx, and vocal tract starts a series of changes that directly influence all methods of alaryngeal speech. An illustration of this anatomical change from before to after laryngectomy is provided in Figure 5-1.

Of critical importance to the topic of postlaryngectomy alaryngeal speech methods is the fact that the person's airway will no longer be linked to other upper airway structures (e.g., the oral cavity), where physiology supports nasal resonance and the articulation of individual speech sounds. In addition, because of the loss of the larynx and its potential to generate sound to support speech, alaryngeal speakers must be instructed to acquire new sources for vocal communication. Although some postlaryngectomy communication methods may use residual biological tissues as a new source of sound generation, others require that an external electronic alaryngeal voicing source be used. Thus, alaryngeal speech options are distinguished as either *intrinsic* or *extrinsic methods of communication* (Doyle, 1994; Graham, 1997; Weinberg, 1982). The term intrinsic indicates that the new sound source is one that is generated by anatomical structures of the body, whereas extrinsic methods rely on some type of external source for voice generation. A brief explanation of each of

---

Box 5-4

Examples, descriptions, and visuals for esophageal, tracheoesophageal, and electronic larynx speech can be found on the WebWhispers website at http://www.webwhispers. org/library/talking-again.asp

---

the three most commonly used methods is provided in the following sections; however, a general understating of normal speech production is necessary first.

Generation of Normal Voice and Speech

To understand how each alaryngeal speech method is achieved, a basic review of the normal voice- and speech-production system is required. A simple physical analog may best illustrate the normal process. For speech to be produced, there must be a power supply, a vibrated sound source, and a filter whereby the source can be modified, modulated, and manipulated into the array of sounds used for any given language. Thus, normal speech involves an aerodynamic power source (the lungs), a structure for the generation of a vibratory sound source or "voice" (the larynx), and a series of anatomical structures that are used to modify that voice source (e.g., the tongue, lips, teeth, jaw, soft palate) for the purpose of speech production.

When a person with a normal system desires to speak, the following process occurs:

- The person takes in a breath and, on expiration, passes air through the larynx, where the vocal folds provide a constriction to that flow of air.

- When expired air passes across the constriction, it creates vibration of the vocal folds.

- The voiced signal subsequently moves into the vocal tract, where it can be shaped via articulators into specific vowel and consonant sounds.

Despite the uniformity of the phonation process already described, the vocal tract is not a fixed size or shape; rather, it can be rapidly and dynamically altered. Changes in the overall length and shape of the vocal tract during speech production enable the voice source to be modified into the unique sounds of speech via an elaborate and coordinated process of articulation. The end result of the preceding and very simplified physical analog is the generation of a speech signal that can be received by a listener during the communication process.

As already mentioned in this chapter, total laryngectomy requires separation of the airway from the upper regions of the vocal tract secondary to surgery. Therefore, not only is the normal voice source lost after laryngectomy, but its power supply and filter are also disconnected from one another. Thus, several factors need to be considered specific to methods of alaryngeal voice and speech, including the source of sound generation and separation of the air supply from regions that were previously involved in normal speech.

Generation of Alaryngeal Voice and Speech

At present, there are three primary options for voice and speech rehabilitation after laryngectomy. These options include esophageal speech, tracheoesophageal speech, and electronic larynx speech, or what is more commonly referred to by clinicians and those who have undergone laryngectomy as use of an electrolarynx (EL) (Box 5-4).

A fourth option, which is powered by air rather than batteries or electricity, is a *pneumatic artificial larynx*; however, it is not widely used relative to the other three options.

TABLE 5-1		
RELATIVE ADVANTAGES AND DISADVANTAGES OF ESOPHAGEAL, TRACHEOESOPHAGEAL, ELECTROLARYNGEAL, AND PNEUMATIC ALARYNGEAL VOICE AND SPEECH METHODS		
ALARYNGEAL VOICE AND SPEECH METHOD	**ADVANTAGES**	**DISADVANTAGES**
Esophageal (intrinsic)	No need for devices; no additional surgery required; can provide a softer, "confidential" level of loudness for private communication	Low pitch; slower speech rate; altered pauses; low relative intensity; difficult to learn for some; requires knowledgeable instruction
Tracheoesophageal (intrinsic)	Higher pitch; increased intensity; near-normal speech rate; quickly acquired in most instances with good instruction	May require a second surgery; requires a prosthetic device that must be maintained and cleaned; may require use of one hand; hygiene issues related to potentially touching stoma; cost of device; irritation of tissue at tracheoesophageal puncture site
Electrolaryngeal (extrinsic)	Easily acquired by most laryngectomees; immediate functional communication can be provided early in rehabilitation; speech is not influenced negatively by stressful communication situations; good loudness, particularly under conditions of background noise; may be better for telephone use	Mechanical and robotic speech quality; potential for mechanical breakdown or loss of battery power; production of a quieter voice is difficult to achieve; requires use of one hand; hygiene issues with intraoral tubes; may not be accepted easily by listeners
Pneumatic (Tokyo) artificial larynx (extrinsic)	Higher pitch relative to other methods; pitch can be modified to some degree by adjusting the vibratory band; relatively normal flow of speech	Devices are not always easily available; ability to couple device to tracheostoma may be somewhat challenging; requires use of at least one hand; hygiene issues with intraoral tube
		Doyle, 1994

Table 5-1 provides a list of the pros and cons of each of these methods. The first two methods, esophageal and tracheoesophageal speech, are intrinsic methods of alaryngeal speech. The remaining two options, the EL and the pneumatic artificial larynx, are extrinsic speech methods because each of them requires an external device to be coupled to the vocal tract to communicate.

Box 5-5

Although the details regarding specific therapeutic methods for teaching and refining esophageal speech are beyond the scope of this chapter, several excellent clinical resources are recommended for those seeking additional information: Doyle (1994, 2005), Graham (1997), Lauder (2012), and Shanks (1994).

As a general rule, extrinsic methods of postlaryngectomy communication are identified broadly as artificial laryngeal or *artificial larynx* speech.

Esophageal Speech

Esophageal speech is a longstanding mode of postlaryngectomy speech (Diedrich, 1968). The term esophageal is used because the new source of voicing is generated by anatomical tissues that generally compose a region at the top of the esophagus. Specifically, the more likely source of esophageal voice is the result of tissues of both the upper esophagus and lower pharynx being set into vibration volitionally (Damste, 1994; Diedrich & Youngstrom, 1966; Doyle, 1994). Thus, this anatomical region is referred to most appropriately as comprising tissues identified as the *pharyngoesophageal (PE) segment*, a band of muscular tissues that forms a merged transitional region related to the esophagus and lower pharynx. As a general rule, the PE segment is a closed ring of muscular tissue (or constriction) when contracted. The area below the segment, the esophagus, can then be considered a relatively open space that serves as a reservoir. The space above it, which forms the lower portion of the pharynx, is also a relatively open structure and can be viewed in a similar manner. Thus, to generate vibration of the PE segment to achieve esophageal voice, the laryngectomee must be taught to move air inferiorly into the esophageal reservoir and then bring that air supply back up through the PE segment to vibrate it and generate esophageal sound (Box 5-5).

Thus, esophageal speakers must be taught to volitionally move air back and forth across the PE segment by actively compressing air within the oral cavity. When a speaker's mouth is closed (i.e., lips are sealed), active compression of the air that is trapped in the oral cavity will increase in pressure to the point at which it will then overcome the muscular force of the PE-segment tissue and push across the segment, filling the esophageal reservoir with air. However, to understand this process and its inherent limitations, some elaboration is necessary.

The amount of air that can be trapped and compressed within the oral cavity is relatively limited (approximately 50 to 80 cc). As such, this power supply is reduced significantly compared to the rather large volumes of air from the lungs (approximately 3,000 to 5,000 cc) that are potentially available to a healthy speaker. Therefore, the esophageal speaker will need to regularly refill the esophagus with air to produce continuous speech. Given the relatively small amounts of air available with each new *insufflation* of air into the esophageal reservoir, esophageal speech may be characterized by the speaker being able to produce only a limited number of syllables on a single air insufflation (Berlin, 1963; Shanks, 1994; Snidecor & Curry, 1959). In addition, because of the limitation in the new esophageal power supply, replenishing air in the esophagus may result in abnormally placed pauses during speech not typically noted in laryngeal speech. This type of alteration in the flow of the speech signal may carry with it an increased demand on the listener. Although the pauses may be brief for excellent esophageal speakers, other esophageal speakers may need to pause and recharge frequently during running speech to maintain esophageal voicing. Thus, the interaction of the new voice source, the PE segment, and the capacity to power it via air captured in the esophageal reservoir serves to distinguish esophageal voice and speech from other methods.

Box 5-6
When the flow of material from the esophagus into the airway via the prosthesis occurs, it is an indication that the prosthesis requires changing, a process that is undertaken by a physician or speech-language pathologist (SLP). In addition, however, leakage that occurs around the prosthesis suggests changes in the integrity of the puncture site itself.

Tracheoesophageal Speech

Tracheoesophageal (TE) speech is another intrinsic method of alaryngeal speech. However, although TE speech also uses the PE segment as the new postlaryngectomy vibratory sound source, its power supply differs from that of the traditional esophageal speaker. First, TE speech is best identified as a surgical-prosthetic method of postlaryngectomy voice rehabilitation. This method was first introduced in 1980 and has been described as "tracheoesophageal puncture (TEP) voice restoration" (Singer & Blom, 1980). For this reason, it is important to acknowledge that TE speech involves a unique surgical procedure that can be performed at the same time as a total laryngectomy (termed a primary TE puncture) or at some point after it (termed a secondary TE puncture). Tracheoesophageal speech also requires the use of a small prosthetic valve that is referred to as a TE puncture voice prosthesis. This TE voice prosthesis does not serve as a new vibratory source but, rather, as a structural conduit or shunt that allows air from the lungs to move into the esophageal reservoir through the pathway provided by the TE puncture and the prosthesis. That air is then used to vibrate the PE segment as a lung-powered or (tracheo)esophageal voice source.

Total laryngectomy creates a separation between the airway and the structures of the vocal tract, so the rationale behind the TE puncture voice-restoration technique was to surgically and prosthetically link these two regions. Anatomically, the trachea sits immediately in front of or anterior to the esophagus and PE segment. Thus, the back wall of the trachea and the front wall of the esophagus are in direct proximity to one another—it is, in fact, a common tissue wall. The TE puncture voice-restoration technique exploits this anatomical relationship by creating a controlled puncture through that common wall. Once the puncture is created, a TE puncture voice prosthesis is then placed within the site. When the tracheostoma is closed, using either a finger or a mechanical pressure-sensitive tracheostoma breathing valve, lung air can be redirected through the prosthesis and into the esophageal reservoir during expiration. In doing so, a laryngectomee who uses TE speech then has access to a more continuous power supply for filling the esophageal reservoir and vibrating the PE segment than would a laryngectomee who uses esophageal speech (Blom, Singer, & Hamaker, 1986; Robbins et al., 1984).

Although a number of different types and sizes of TE puncture voice prostheses are commercially available, all of them are considered one-way valves or prosthetic shunts. That is, the TE puncture voice prosthesis was designed to allow air from the lungs to move easily through the prosthesis and then into the esophageal reservoir; however, its design also was structured to resist movement of material from the esophagus through the prosthesis and into the airway. This one-way valve serves to reduce the potential for contents of the esophagus (e.g., saliva, liquids, food) to move through the valve into the airway, where aspiration can occur. Despite the fact that the airway and vocal tract are separated as a result of total laryngectomy, the airway still must be protected because of the potential for the contents of the esophagus to flow backward into the TE puncture voice prosthesis (Box 5-6).

Thus, TE puncture voice prostheses were designed to be minimally resistant to airflow from the lungs into the esophagus but maximally resistant to flow in the opposite direction. Overall, TE puncture voice restoration involves a number of complex issues that require careful assessment for candidacy, a considerable understanding of this alaryngeal method, and an ability to troubleshoot difficulties with its implementation (Lewin, 2005) (Case Study 5-1).

CASE STUDY 5-1

PATIENT NAME: ANNE

Clinical Status: 2 years 8 months after laryngectomy

Anne is a 73-year-old married woman who underwent total laryngectomy 32 months ago after a diagnosis of squamous cell carcinoma that was found to have crossed the anterior commissure of the larynx. At that time, she also underwent a bilateral neck dissection followed by a 6-week course of adjuvant RT. Her postsurgery and postradiation recovery was uneventful. On the basis of self-report, she is currently in good health and is active socially.

In the period immediately after her total laryngectomy, as well as through the period of RT, Anne communicated with an EL. She became a very proficient user of a neck-type device. With the exception of the mechanical quality of the EL signal, it met her communication needs fully, and no restrictions were noted. However, 7 months after her laryngectomy, Anne received instruction in esophageal speech. With instruction, she quickly acquired very good esophageal speech that she then began to use as her primary method of communication. Anne reported, however, that the lowered intensity of her esophageal speech has created some challenges in specific settings; in those instances, she is not hesitant to use the EL. However, in recent months, the reduced intensity of her esophageal speech has created increased communication difficulties for her when interacting with same-aged peers who have some level of hearing loss. For this reason, Anne is now seeking information on a secondary TE puncture from her otolaryngologist and SLP.

Anne's primary rationale for seeking information on TE puncture voice restoration is based on her lack of loudness when using esophageal speech. Although she still uses the EL successfully, she feels that the mechanical robot-like quality results in the loss of a feminine voice quality that she does not experience when using esophageal speech; this change is somewhat bothersome to her. By undergoing TE puncture voice restoration, Anne believes that her loudness will improve and that it will facilitate better communication with her friends and family.

In consulting with her health care providers, the decision to undergo a secondary TE puncture was made. Because Anne has excellent esophageal speech despite its reduced intensity, the SLP reasoned that a similar quality is likely to exist after the puncture. This reasoning is based on the fact that the same intrinsic tissues are used for both esophageal and TE voice generation. In addition, because of the access to pulmonary air, Anne's TE voice would be louder, which will make her interactions with others who may exhibit reductions in hearing less problematic. Finally, both her surgeon and SLP acknowledged that should the TE puncture fail for whatever reason, Anne would still be able to use the other alaryngeal methods without considerable risk of a change in her communication success. Although concerns related to the expense of the TE puncture voice prosthesis and general issues related to its management are a slight concern to Anne, they do not seem to override the advantages she sees in seeking a TE puncture.

Artificial Electrolarynx Speech

The electronic artificial larynx has a long history in postlaryngectomy rehabilitation (Keith, Shanks, & Doyle, 2005). It is unfortunate that, over the years, the EL has been met with some unwarranted negative bias against its use (Berry, 1978; Doyle, 1994; Duguay, 1978; Gates et al., 1982). However, at the very least, the EL is likely to serve as an important first step in speech rehabilitation after laryngectomy and to be used for at least some communication purposes by more than half of all laryngectomees 2 years after surgery (Meltzner et al., 2005). The EL is an extrinsic method of alaryngeal speech that is designed to provide an electronically powered external voice source. In addition, the EL may be used by a speaker in two different ways. First, and most commonly, the EL can be placed directly on tissues of the neck, the chin, or the cheek. When the EL is activated by the user manually, the EL signal is transferred across that tissue into the vocal tract, where it can be articulated into the sounds of speech. When the EL is used in this manner, it is referred to as a transcervical or neck-type EL. In contrast, the second method of using an EL is achieved by introducing the signal into the oral cavity. Some EL devices are designed to have a small tube attached to the device. Thus, the EL sound source can be transferred through the tube and introduced directly into the oral cavity, where it can then be articulated into the sounds of speech. When this approach is used, it is termed a transoral or mouth-type EL. It is important to note that for some commercial neck-type EL devices, an adapter also may be used to convert such devices for intraoral use. This adapter simply attaches to the portion of the EL that would be applied to the neck and allows a small-diameter oral tube to be inserted into that adapter. Regardless of the method of EL use, instruction by a qualified SLP serves to optimize communication outcomes and the efficiency of this mode of alaryngeal speech (Doyle, 1994, 2005) (Case Study 5-2).

Although there are no published data on the relative proportion of laryngectomees who use either a neck-type or an intraoral EL device for communication purposes, clinical observation suggests that the neck-type EL is used more commonly. Regardless of whether one chooses to use a neck-type or intraoral type of EL, limitations exist, and both approaches entail important clinical considerations. For example, in the early postoperative period, intraoral devices are preferred, because contact with tissues of the neck after surgery should be avoided to reduce discomfort. Similarly, a neck-type EL device may not be effective in those who experience considerable swelling of the tissues of the neck as a result of postsurgical fluid retention (i.e., lymphedema) or in those who have less compliant tissues or fibrosis as a result of the effects of radiotherapy or a combination of these factors. Both of these conditions, as well as factors related to scarring, sensitivity, pain, etc., and problems with manual dexterity may limit the potential effectiveness of both neck-type and intraoral EL devices. That said, intraoral devices may have limitations associated with reduced articulation accuracy because of placement of the intraoral tube directly into the oral cavity. Although clinical instruction on the use of the intraoral EL typically directs the patient to place the tube toward one corner of the mouth, placement may reduce tongue movement and, consequently, articulatory precision and intelligibility (Doyle, 2005).

These challenges are some of the most obvious concerns relative to use of the EL. However, it must be noted that EL instruction should be a primary part of all postlaryngectomy communication rehabilitation programs. At the very least, instruction in EL use enables those who are in the early days and weeks after surgery to communicate their basic wants and needs at a critical point in the recovery and rehabilitation process. It is recommended, therefore, that all laryngectomees be introduced to the EL, particularly an intraoral type of device, in the early period after surgery. Instruction by the SLP should be directed toward the basics of device operation, determining its correct placement, manipulating it to maintain correct placement, and use of a slowed speech rate with overarticulation of speech sounds. Brief periods of training often garner substantial benefits for not only laryngectomees but also members of their family and the team of health care providers who work with them over the short- and long-term trajectory of their treatment and recovery. The ability to communicate early in the process, even with just single words or short phrases, is an important factor in facilitating positive outcomes.

Pneumatic Artificial Larynx—the "Tokyo" Device

By broadening the category of extrinsic options, less frequently used approaches that may rely on an external vibratory source that is powered by the laryngectomized speaker's lung air can be

---

CASE STUDY 5-2

PATIENT NAME: DANIEL

Clinical Status: 8 days after laryngectomy

Daniel is a 66-year-old retired postal worker and veteran who underwent laryngectomy and unilateral neck dissection 8 days ago. His first diagnosis of LC was made approximately 1 year earlier after intermittent voice changes and ear pain over the previous 6 months. At the time of initial diagnosis, a small well-defined squamous cell carcinoma was identified on his left vocal fold. He received 31 sessions of radiation; however, he was recently diagnosed with a recurrence that necessitated the total laryngectomy. Eight days after surgery, he has been declared medically stable, and follow-up with an SLP has been requested. It is anticipated that he will be discharged home in several days.

He has been communicating for the last 4 days by simply writing in a notebook. Because of the recent surgery and the status of his postsurgical neck, the SLP introduces an intraoral EL to Daniel. During this initial postoperative consultation, Daniel is informed about the basic operation of the EL. The SLP informs Daniel that she will place and operate the device initially but then allow him to try to use it with instruction. The SLP operates the on-off control of the intraoral EL, and preliminary instructions are provided to Daniel so that he works to slow his articulation and speak in a deliberate fashion, attempting to overarticulate the speech materials that are presented to him for repetition.

During this session, the SLP also works to place the intraoral tube in the best possible position within the oral cavity without disrupting tongue movement during speech. The SLP has identified a position lateral to the tip of Daniel's tongue, at an insertion depth of approximately 1 inch. Again, the clinician reiterates the instructions for a slowed speech rate with overarticulation. Reasonable success with basic phrases, yes-no responses, and his ability to say his name and make several other requests is achieved relatively quickly in this session.

The SLP next instructs Daniel on how to hold the device and operate the on-off button. Then, using a mirror, she instructs Daniel on the best location for tube placement. The next task focuses on having Daniel operate the device with the tube in a fixed position that rests against his lower teeth. The SLP continues to provide ongoing instruction, encouraging Daniel to turn the EL on before he wishes to speak and then leaving it on until he finishes. She informs him that they will work on refining on-off control in later sessions.

The clinician ends the session by reviewing all issues that were addressed during the session and providing him with a simple list of instructions. She asks if he would like her to leave the device with him, and he agrees. However, the SLP encouraged him to also use the writing pad if others are having difficulty understanding him. She indicated to Daniel that she would return the next morning to continue work on the tasks she has presented and on some new goals.

---

considered. One option involves the use of a pneumatic artificial larynx, a device through which lung air, passing freely from the tracheostoma, is directed through a coupler that houses a reed-type vibratory device. This device is termed a Tokyo artificial larynx (Keith, Shanks, & Doyle, 2005; Weinberg & Riekena, 1972). As the laryngectomee exhales, air moves through the housing, the reed vibrates, and that sound source is directed via a flexible tube into the patient's oral cavity, where it can be articulated into speech. Thus, although the power supply differs, the introduction of the alaryngeal voiced signal into the vocal tract is similar to that from an intraoral EL. As a consequence, concerns related to placement and potential inference with articulatory movement also exist with this method.

LIMITATIONS ASSOCIATED WITH ALARYNGEAL VOICE AND SPEECH

Having options relative to verbal communication after laryngectomy is important on several levels. First, multiple options provide a greater chance that one of them will provide a functional and acceptable means of alaryngeal communication to the laryngectomee. Second, because of their relative advantages and disadvantages, some options may be preferred by patients on the basis of their own particular communicative needs (e.g., environmental concerns, type of vocation or avocational activities). Clinical research has found that communication disability secondary to the use of alaryngeal voice and speech is highly variable both within and across the three most widely used modes—esophageal, TE, and electrolaryngeal speech (Cox & Doyle, 2014; Eadie et al., 2012; Eadie & Doyle, 2004; Moukarbel et al., 2011; Oridate et al., 2009;).

The best postlaryngectomy communication outcomes will almost certainly be achieved if the laryngectomee is well informed about all of these methods and their relative limitations. Decisions made by professionals alone without consultation with the laryngectomee, regardless of how well intentioned, are more likely to result in an unfavorable outcome. Yet, one issue is perfectly clear: there is no one perfect alaryngeal speech method.

The most promising approach to restoring verbal communication after total laryngectomy ultimately should be focused on effectively meeting the communication needs of each individual. Similarly, there are no data to suggest that multiple communication methods cannot be used. For example, someone who has gained proficiency with either esophageal speech or TE puncture voice restoration may also choose to use an EL in particular situations. Using one alaryngeal method does not in any way limit one's ability to use another; in fact, having the ability to use two communication methods proficiently has substantial advantages for many reasons.

Regardless of the method used, it is important to understand that the differences across the three methods described here are relative. In addition, there is the very important issue of individual differences. Despite a rather large body of clinical data over many years that includes a variety of acoustic and auditory-perceptual assessments of alaryngeal voice and speech, there is no such thing as a typical or average laryngectomee. Each laryngectomy surgery is unique, as is each laryngectomee. Those who undergo total laryngectomy can present with a variety of issues that cross both anatomical (structural) and physiological (functioning) lines, and these issues collectively influence their capacity and proficiency with postlaryngectomy speech.

Many emerging issues will likely create additional challenges to postlaryngectomy rehabilitation in the future. Factors might include the extent of surgical reconstruction and the potential need for flap reconstruction approaches to compensate for large surgical defects when LC is more extensive. In such instances, surgical excision may extend into the pharynx and beyond. In those for whom, in addition to total laryngectomy, there is a need for partial or total removal of the tongue (*glossectomy*), the impact of such changes on speech may be dramatic, and their effects on quality of life may be devastating.

COMMUNICATION CHALLENGES

All methods of alaryngeal speech are identified by listeners as non-normal in terms of signal quality. As a result, these changes may reduce the effectiveness of a patient's communication in the following important ways:

- Auditory-perceptual judgments of alaryngeal speech indicate that listeners are sensitive to its alterations of frequency (pitch), intensity (loudness), and overall character (quality).

  ○ With some methods, and depending on the proficiency of the speaker, very obvious changes in the rate of speech also may be observed, which might influence a listener's over-all assessment of a person's alaryngeal speech (Bennett & Weinberg, 1973; Doyle & Eadie, 2005; Eadie & Doyle, 2005a, 2005b).

A total laryngectomy may result in a variety of other changes, including the following, that directly and significantly influence one's speech and communication capabilities in the broadest sense:

- Mobility of the tongue and jaw may be reduced.

- A decrease in saliva may negatively influence the precision of articulation.

- Changes in resonance may be noted.

- Physical changes that are a consequence of surgery and are highly visible to the communica-tive partner may create discomfort during such interactions.

Overall, there is a considerable body of literature that shows that alaryngeal speech methods may be less intelligible to listeners (Doyle, Danhauer, & Reed, 1988; Holley et al., 1983; McCroskey & Mulligan, 1963; Weiss & Basili, 1985). However, despite such limitations secondary to the acquisition of a new postlaryngectomy voice, many laryngectomees are able to communicate quite effectively in a variety of settings.

Clearly, instruction by professionals with the objective of optimizing all aspects of the patient's communication is essential. Peer support, through Lost Chord or New Voice clubs or other laryn-gectomee support groups, in addition to online resources, may also be of great value as patients move through the rehabilitation process. Several online resources that can provide valuable infor-mation to the laryngectomee and members of his or her family include the following:

- WebWhispers (http://www.webwhispers.org/index.asp)

- International Association of Laryngectomees (http://www.theial.com/ial/)

- Speech Therapy Toolbox website (www.speechtherapytoolbox.com/laryngectomy.html)

Regardless of whether one uses esophageal speech, undergoes TE puncture voice restoration, or chooses to use any type of artificial larynx or EL, a program of systematic instruction will serve to maximize that person's communication potential. Therefore, careful consideration and ongo-ing discussion between the laryngectomee and his or her SLP must occur to evaluate the relative advantages and disadvantages of each communication method, the specific communication needs and environments of the laryngectomee (e.g., telephone use at work, presence of background noise, avocational needs), and the potential duration of treatment. In addition, the various expectations of the current health care systems may also need to be addressed, in that particular centers may dictate "choice" in the current practice environment. For example, limitations in operating room time may result in a decision by some centers to encourage and simultaneously complete a TE puncture at the time of one's laryngectomy (i.e., a primary TE puncture). Similarly, those who are treated in larger centers may have access to an array of clinicians with broader levels of expertise in all modes of alaryngeal speech rehabilitation. Such enhancements in clinician expertise may eliminate bias in the information provided to those who have undergone a laryngectomy (Doyle, 1994). Finally, a frank discussion related to issues of how listeners may perceive and react to all ala-ryngeal voice and speech methods is essential, because a non-normal voicing source may influence overall communication effectiveness in some instances. Counseling related to postlaryngectomy communication options is always best served through an honest and open discussion between the laryngectomee and the clinician about how others may respond to the unusual nature of alaryngeal speech, the potential for a listener's discomfort in participating in communication, and the social and emotional impact of such communication challenges.

It is equally important to provide those who will undergo total laryngectomy with information that carefully identifies the types of changes that will occur. Being able to make an informed decision is essential for achieving the best level of patient care. Similarly, for those who have undergone laryngectomy, clear and straightforward information about communication challenges should be addressed directly and with compassion. The SLP is likely to serve as the patient's best advocate by providing information on and addressing communication challenges, gathering information for the patient, and assisting with the interpretation of a vast array of information, as appropriate (Doyle, 1994). Through these types of advocacy, the laryngectomee can become more comfortable in expressing his or her concerns, identifying problems, and, perhaps just as important, actively engaging with the clinician in problem solving.

CONCLUSION

Because laryngectomy results in the loss of the primary structure for the generation of voice, the larynx, there exists the need to restore verbal communication with a new alaryngeal method of speech. This need can be satisfied with the three most commonly used alaryngeal methods—esophageal speech, TE speech, and electrolaryngeal speech—and the pneumatic artificial (Tokyo) larynx. Although each method provides a suitable option for many laryngectomees, no perfect method exists. There are specific advantages and disadvantages associated with each of these methods. However, with a focus being placed on achieving the best possible communication in the period of early recovery, and in the shorter- and longer-term period of rehabilitation, one must consider the specific needs of each patient. Each of the methods described in this chapter provides a viable option that can meet the communicative needs of many patients. Although none of these alaryngeal methods is without limitations, careful consideration of each one of them, along with structured and systematic instruction by a trained SLP, will facilitate the greatest likelihood of success.

REFERENCES

Bennett, S., & Weinberg, B. (1973). Acceptability ratings of normal, esophageal, and artificial larynx speech. *Journal of Speech and Hearing Research, 16,* 608–615.

Berlin, C. I. (1963). Clinical measurement of esophageal speech: I. Methodology and curves of skill acquisition. *Journal of Speech and Hearing Disorders, 28*(1), 42–51.

Berry, W. R. (1978). Attitudes of speech langu3age pathologists and otolaryngologists about artificial larynges. In S. J. Salmon & L. P. Goldstein (Eds.), *The artificial larynx handbook.* New York, NY: Grune & Stratton.

Bjordal, K., Freng, A., Thorvik, J., & Kaasa, S. (1995). Patient self-reported and clinician-rated quality of life in head and neck cancer patients: A cross-sectional study. *European Journal of Cancer and Oral Oncology, 31,* 235–241.

Blom, E. D., Singer, M. I., & Hamaker, R. C. (1986). A prospective study of tracheoesophageal speech. *Archives of Otolaryngology–Head and Neck Surgery, 112,* 440–447.

Blood, G. W., Luther, A. R., & Stemple, J. C. (1992). Coping and adjustment in alaryngeal speakers. *American Journal of Speech-Language Pathology, 1,* 63–69.

Brown, S. I., & Doyle, P. C. (1999). The woman who is laryngectomized: Parallels, perspectives, and a reevaluation of practice. *Journal of Speech-Language Pathology and Audiology, 23,* 10–15.

Clements, K. S., Rassekh, C. H., Seikaly, H., Hokanson, J. A., & Calhoun, K. H. (1997). Communication after laryngectomy: An assessment of patient satisfaction. *Archives of Otolaryngology–Head and Neck Surgery, 123,* 493–496.

Cox, S. R., & Doyle, P. C. (2014). The influence of electrolarynx use on postlaryngectomy voice-related quality of life. *Otolaryngology–Head and Neck Surgery, 150,* 1005-1009.

Cox, S. R., Theurer, J. A., Spaulding, S. J., & Doyle, P. C. (2015). The multidimensional impact of total laryngectomy on women. *Journal of Communication Disorders, 56,* 59-75.

Damste, P. H. (1994). Some obstacles in learning esophageal speech. In R. L. Keith & F. L. Darley (Eds.), *Laryngectomy rehabilitation.* San Diego, CA: College-Hill Press.

Diedrich, W. M. (1968). The mechanism of esophageal speech. *Annals of the New York Academy of Sciences, 155,* 303-317.

Diedrich, W. M., & Youngstrom, K. A. (1966). *Alaryngeal speech.* Springfield, IL: Charles C. Thomas.

Doyle, P. C. (1994). *Foundations of voice and speech rehabilitation following laryngeal cancer.* San Diego, CA: Singular.

Doyle, P. C. (2005). Clinical procedures for training use of the electronic artificial larynx. In P. C. Doyle & R. L. Keith (Eds.), *Contemporary considerations in the treatment and rehabilitation of head and neck cancer: Voice, speech, and swallowing.* Austin, TX: Pro-Ed.

Doyle, P. C., Danhauer, J. L., & Reed, C. G. (1988). Listeners' perceptions of consonants produced by esophageal and tracheoesophageal talkers. *Journal of Speech and Hearing Disorders, 53,* 400-407.

Doyle, P. C., & Eadie, T. L. (2005). The perceptual nature of alaryngeal voice and speech. In P. C. Doyle & R. L. Keith (Eds.). *Contemporary considerations in the treatment and rehabilitation of head and neck cancer: Voice, speech, and swallowing* (pp. 113-140). Austin, TX: Pro-Ed.

Duguay, M. J. (1978). Why not both? In S. J. Salmon & L. P. Goldstein (Eds.), *The artificial larynx handbook.* New York, NY: Grune & Stratton.

Eadie, T. L., Day, A. M., Sawin, D. E., Lamvik, K., & Doyle, P. C. (2012). Auditory-perceptual speech outcomes and quality of life after total laryngectomy. *Otolaryngology–Head and Neck Surgery, 148*(1), 82-88. doi:10.1177/0194599812461755.

Eadie, T. L., & Doyle, P. C. (2004). Auditory-perceptual scaling and quality of life in tracheoesophageal speakers. *The Laryngoscope, 114*(4), 753-759.

Eadie, T. L., & Doyle, P. C. (2005a). Quality of life in male tracheoesophageal (TE) speakers. *Journal of Rehabilitation Research and Development, 42,* 115-124.

Eadie, T. L., & Doyle, P. C. (2005b). Scaling of pleasantness and acceptability in tracheoesophageal (TE) speakers. *Journal of Voice, 19,* 373-383.

Eadie, T. L., Day, A. M. B., Sawin, D. E., Lamvik, K., & Doyle, P. C. (2012). Auditory-perceptual speech outcomes and quality of life after total laryngectomy. *Otolaryngology–Head and Neck Surgery, 148,* 82-88.

Eadie, T. L., Doyle, P. C., Hansen, K., & Beaudin, P. G. (2008). Influence of speaker gender on listener judgements of tracheoesophageal speech. *Journal of Voice, 22,* 43-57.

Finizia, C., Hammerlid, E., Westin, T., & Lindström, J. (1998). Quality of life and voice in patients with laryngeal carcinoma: A posttreatment comparison of laryngectomy (salvage surgery) versus radiotherapy. *Laryngoscope, 108,* 1566-1573.

Forastiere, A. A., Goepfert, H., Maor, M., Pajak, T. F., Weber, R., Morrison, W., ... Cooper, J. (2003). Concurrent chemotherapy and radiotherapy for organ preservation in advanced laryngeal cancer. *New England Journal of Medicine, 349,* 2091-2098.

Gates, G., Ryan, W., Cooper, J., Lawlis, G., Cantu, E., Hyashi, T., ... Hearne, E. (1982). Current status of laryngectomee rehabilitation: I. Results of therapy. *American Journal of Otolaryngology, 3,* 1-17.

Gotay, C. C., & Moore, T. D. (1992). Assessing quality of life in head and neck cancer. *Quality of Life Research, 11,* 5-17.

Graham, M. S. (1997). *The clinician's guide to alaryngeal speech therapy.* Waltham, MA: Butterworth-Heinemann.

Graham, M. S., & Palmer, A. (2002). Gender difference considerations for individuals with laryngectomies. *Contemporary Issues in Communication Sciences and Disorders, 29,* 59-67.

Hanna, E., Sherman, A., Cash, D., Adams, D., Vural, E., Fan, C. Y., & Suen, J. Y. (2004). Quality of life for patients following total laryngectomy vs chemoradiation for laryngeal preservation. *Archives of Otolaryngology–Head and Neck Surgery, 130,* 875-879.

Hassan, S. J., & Weymuller, E. A. (1993). Assessment of quality of life in head and neck cancer patients. *Head and Neck, 15,* 485-496.

Hilgers, F. J. M., & Ackerstaff, A. H. (2005). Respiratory consequences of total laryngectomy and the need for pulmonary protection and rehabilitation. In P. C. Doyle & R. L. Keith (Eds.), *Contemporary considerations in the treatment and rehabilitation of head and neck cancer: Voice, speech, and swallowing* (pp. 503-520). Austin, TX: Pro-Ed.

Hillman, R. E., Walsh, M. J., Wolf, G. T., Fisher, S. G., & Hong, W. K. (1998). Functional outcomes following treatment for advanced laryngeal cancer. Part I—Voice preservation in advanced laryngeal cancer. Part II—Laryngectomy rehabilitation: The state of the art in the VA System. Research Speech-Language Pathologists. Department of Veterans Affairs Laryngeal Cancer Study Group. *Annals of Otology, Rhinology, and Laryngology Supplement, 172,* 1-27.

Holley, S., Lerman, J., & Randolph, K. (1983). A comparison of the intelligibility of esophageal, electrolaryngeal, and normal speech in quiet and in noise. *Journal of Communication Disorders, 16*, 143–155.

Karnell, L. H., Funk, G. F., & Hoffman, H. T. (2000). Assessing head and neck cancer patient outcome domains. *Head and Neck, 22*, 6–11.

Keith, R. L., Shanks, J. C., & Doyle, P. C. (2005). Historical highlights: Laryngectomy rehabilitation. In P. C. Doyle & R. L. Keith (Eds.), *Contemporary considerations in the treatment and rehabilitation of head and neck cancer: Voice, speech and swallowing.* Austin, TX: Pro-Ed.

Lauder, E. (2012). *Self-help for the laryngectomee.* San Antonio, TX: Lauder Publishing.

Lewin, J. S. (2005). Problems associated with alaryngeal speech. In P. C. Doyle & R. L. Keight (Eds.), *Contemporary considerations in the treatment of head and neck cancer: Voice, speech, and swallowing.* Austin, TX: Pro-Ed.

McCroskey, R. L., & Mulligan, M. (1963). The relative intelligibility of esophageal speech and artificial-larynx speech. *Journal of Speech and Hearing Disorders, 28*, 37–41.

Meltzner, G., Hillman, R. E., Heaton, J. T., Houston, K. M., Kobler, J., & Qi, Y. (2005). Electrolaryngeal speech: The state of the art and future directions for development. In P. C. Doyle & R. L. Keith (Eds.), *Contemporary considerations in the treatment of head and neck cancer: Voice, speech, and swallowing.* Austin, TX: Pro-Ed.

Mendenhall, W. M., Morris, C. G., Stringer, S. P., Amdur, R. J., Hinerman, R. W., Villaret, D. B., & Robbins, K. T. (2002). Voice rehabilitation after total laryngectomy and postoperative radiation therapy. *Journal of Clinical Oncology, 20*, 2500–2505.

Moukarbel, R. V., Doyle, P. C., Yoo, J., Franklin, J. H., Fung, K., & Day, A. (2011). Voice-related quality of life (V-RQOL) outcomes in laryngectomees. *Head and Neck, 33*, 31–36.

Oridate, N., Homma, A., Suzuki, S., Nakamaru, Y., Suzuki, F., Hatakeyama, H., … Fukuda, S. (2009). Voice-related quality of life after treatment of laryngeal cancer. *Archives of Otolaryngology–Head and Neck Surgery, 135*, 363–368.

Robbins, J., Fisher, H. B., Blom, E. C., & Singer, M. I. (1984). A comparative acoustic study of normal, esophageal, and tracheoesophageal speech production. *Journal of Speech and Hearing Disorders, 49*, 202–210.

Robertson, S. M., Yeo, J. C. L., Sabey, L., Young, D., & MacKenzie, K. (2013). Effects of tumor staging and treatment modality on functional outcome and quality of life after treatment for laryngeal cancer. *Head and Neck, 35*, 1759–1763.

Salmon, S. J. (2005). Commonalities among alaryngeal speech methods. In P.C. Doyle & R. L. Keith (Eds.), *Contemporary considerations in the treatment and rehabilitation of head and neck cancer: Voice, speech, and swallowing.* Austin, TX: Pro-Ed.

Searl, J. P., & Small, L. H. (2002). Gender and masculinity-femininity ratings of tracheoesophageal speech. *Journal of Communication Disorders, 35*, 407–420.

Shanks, J. C. (1994). Developing esophageal communication. In R.L. Keith & F.L. Darley (Eds.), *Laryngectomee rehabilitation* (pp. 205–217). Austin, TX: Pro-Ed.

Shipp, T. (1967). Frequency, duration and perceptual measures in relation to judgments of alaryngeal speech acceptability. *Journal of Speech and Hearing Research, 10*, 417–427.

Silver, C. E., Beitler, J. J., Shaha, A. R., Rinaldo, A., & Ferlito, A. (2009). Current trends in initial management of laryngeal cancer: The declining use of open surgery. *European Archives of Oto-Rhino-Laryngology, 266*, 1333–1352.

Singer, M. I., & Blom, E. D. (1980). An endoscopic technique for restoration of voice after laryngectomy. *Annals of Otology, Rhinology, and Laryngology, 89*, 529–533.

Snidecor, J. C., & Curry, E. T. (1959). Temporal and pitch aspects of superior esophageal speech. *Annals of Otology, Rhinology, and Laryngology, 68*, 623–629.

Timmermans, A. J., de Gooijer, C. J., Hamming-Vrieze, O., Hilgers, F. J. M., & van den Brekel, M. W. M. (2014). T3-T4 laryngeal cancer in the Netherlands Cancer Institute: 10-year results of the consistent application of an organ-preserving/-sacrificing protocol. *Head and Neck, 37*, 1495–1505.

Trudeau, M. D., & Qi, Y. Y. (1990). Acoustic characteristics of female tracheoesophageal speech. *Journal of Speech and Hearing Disorders, 55*, 244–250.

Weinberg, B. (1982). Speech after laryngectomy: An overview and review of acoustic and temporal characteristics of esophageal speech. In A. Sekey (Ed.), *Electroacoustic analysis and enhancement of alaryngeal speech* (pp. 5–48). Springfield, IL: Charles C. Thomas.

Weinberg, B., & Riekena, A. (1973). Speech produced with the Tokyo artificial larynx. *Journal of Speech and Hearing Disorders, 38*(3), 383–389.

Weiss, M. S., & Basili, A. M. (1985). Electrolaryngeal speech produced by laryngectomized subjects: Perceptual characteristics. *Journal of Speech and Hearing Research, 28*, 294–300.

Williams, S. E., & Watson, J. B. (1985). Differences in speaking proficiencies in three laryngectomee groups. *Archives of Otolaryngology–Head & Neck Surgery, 111*, 216.

6

Nutrition and Swallowing Challenges in Laryngeal Cancer

Rachael E. Kammer, MS, CCC-SLP, BCS-S and
Tessa Goldsmith, MA, CCC-SLP

The larynx is a multiuse structure that is responsible for guarding the airway during swallowing, opening for respiration, and regulating airflow for phonation, whereas the esophagus is a critical passageway for food into the stomach. Because the larynx is adjacent to the esophagus, food material may effectively "go down the wrong tube" and enter the trachea, rather than the esophagus, when the laryngeal structures that protect the airway are removed or compromised. When laryngeal airway protection consistently fails, food material may pass into the airway and result in a decline in health or even death. By invading the neural, muscular, and cartilaginous substrates of the larynx, laryngeal tumors can negatively affect airway protection. Surgery, radiation therapy, and chemotherapy may also alter the laryngeal structures that function to protect the airway during swallowing. In addition, because of the proximity of the larynx to the esophagus, laryngeal tumors and treatment for them may have secondary negative effects on the structure and function of the cervical esophagus that result in swallowing dysfunction (i.e., dysphagia).

In this chapter, the nature of dysphagia in patients with laryngeal cancer (LC) across different laryngeal tumor subsites and after a variety of treatment options (i.e., radiation, chemotherapy, surgery) across the continuum of care from diagnosis to delayed treatment effects is presented. We also discuss how eradicated tumors do not restore laryngeal function to baseline status because treatment effects may create as many issues with swallowing as the diseased state can. Late radiation effects, regardless of whether surgery or chemotherapy is involved, can cause significant problems with airway protection, even in patients with early-stage disease.

Friberg, J. C., & Vinney, L. A.
Laryngeal Cancer: An Interdisciplinary
Resource for Practitioners (pp. 91-110).
© 2017 Taylor and Francis Group.

Box 6-1

HORIZONTAL AND VERTICAL PLANES OF AIRWAY PROTECTION

Airway protection can be viewed as a two-dimensional process:

1. Contraction of the intrinsic laryngeal musculature during swallowing provides a horizontal level of closure of the larynx. Specifically, this sequence progresses as follows:

   - The arytenoid cartilages rotate and rock forward to contact the petiole of the epiglottis.
   - The true and false vocal folds adduct, which closes the glottis.
   - The epiglottis deflects as a function of laryngeal rise and tongue-base retraction.

2. The vertical level of airway protection occurs as the suprahyoid muscles, especially the geniohyoid and mylohyoid muscles, distract the entire larynx away from the posterior pharyngeal wall, tucking it under the tongue and opening the pharyngoesophageal junction to allow passage of the bolus into the cervical esophagus.

AIRWAY-PROTECTION CONSIDERATIONS

Accurate diagnosis and comprehensive management of dysphagia after LC and its treatment demand a robust understanding of the coordination between airway protection by the larynx with the opening of the cervical esophagus. The former function prevents food material from entering the airway, and the latter allows food to move into the stomach for proper nutrition. Both functions must occur simultaneously to promote adequate nutrition and prevent infection in the respiratory system. When food material enters the larynx but does not descend below the true vocal folds, *penetration* has occurred. When this material passes between the true vocal folds, aspiration has occurred. To facilitate relevant and effective treatment, the mechanism that is causing the swallowing dysfunction must be identified and well understood.

Airway protection can be thought of as occurring in both the horizontal and vertical planes, wherein the anatomy of the larynx acts in separate yet functional ways (Box 6-1). It is this redundancy that provides an enhanced safeguard of the airway in case one mechanism is faulty. This redundancy in airway protection may permit safe swallowing of material with a viscous consistency even in the case of vocal fold paralysis from laryngeal tumor resection that causes the glottis to remain open during swallowing.

As discussed in Chapter 1, cancers that originate in the larynx but progress to extralaryngeal structures, such as the posterior pharyngeal wall and the pyriform sinuses, can cause deficiencies in bolus clearance. Specifically, when masses in the supraglottis extend into the base of the tongue, liquids and especially solid foods may accumulate in the vallecular space and pyriform sinuses after the swallow. Hyolaryngeal excursion (the elevation and anterior movement of the entire laryngeal complex by way of contraction of the suprahyoid muscles) and *epiglottic inversion* (the downward movement of the epiglottis over the laryngeal vestibule) are likely to be impaired via the presence of such tumors. Early- and late-stage laryngeal tumors may invade the aryepiglottic folds, the epiglottis, and the ventricular folds by stenting open the laryngeal vestibule and/or inhibiting retroflexion of the epiglottis. In addition, large-volume tumors can obstruct the airway and cause stridor and shortness of breath.

The treatment of laryngeal tumors can further compromise swallow function and therefore affect airway protection. Specifically, after radiotherapy, sensory changes can impact the speed

---

BOX 6-2

Adjuvant radiation therapy is applied after initial surgical management in an effort to eradicate microscopic disease that cannot be resected. It serves to increase likelihood of cure.

---

and agility with which the pharyngeal swallow response is elicited and can result in the following problems:

- Penetration of liquids into the larynx before the onset of hyolaryngeal elevation
- Aspiration during the swallow if vocal fold adduction and closure of the laryngeal vestibule are delayed or incomplete
- Aspiration after the swallow from material that has accumulated in the larynx as the system returns to rest
- Residual material from the valleculae and pyriform sinuses spills into the larynx and trachea after the swallow as a result of associated pharyngeal dysfunction

As important as sensory awareness of the bolus before and during the swallow is, the sensation of bolus entry into the trachea after the swallow is even more important. LCs at all levels of involvement can result in sensory loss and, thus, *silent aspiration*. The phenomenon of silent aspiration is the result of limited sensory feedback from the laryngeal, pharyngeal, and subglottic regions. Silent aspiration is especially problematic; because the person cannot sense material moving between and below the vocal folds, no attempt is made to clear the material via coughing. In some cases, a patient may eventually cough in response to large-volume airway invasion and, provided the patient is able to expectorate the majority of the aspirated material, no significant pulmonary sequelae may ensue. In contrast, if the material is not cleared via cough or no attempt to expectorate the material is made, serious consequences, such as *aspiration pneumonia*, may result.

TREATMENT DECISIONS AND FUNCTIONAL OUTCOMES FOR SWALLOWING

The algorithm for treating early-stage, low-volume, and localized cancers of the supraglottic and glottic larynx (typically stage T1 or T2 lesions) is clear: a single modality, either surgery or radiation therapy alone, results in an excellent prognosis for survival. The treatment goal is curative with the expectation that laryngeal function will be preserved for both voice and swallowing. Supportive care during treatment is limited to pain control, management of secretions, and post-surgical care. Most patients with stage T1 or T2 tumors in the absence of *lymphadenopathy* (abnormal swelling of the lymph nodes) do not require feeding through a *gastrostomy tube* (G-tube).

Until the 1990s, advanced LCs were treated with surgery, including total laryngectomy, and adjuvant radiation therapy (Box 6-2). Functional swallowing was preserved in these patients, but their voice was sacrificed and their quality of life was complicated by the presence of a tracheostoma (McNeil, 1981). The optimal treatment approach has proven to be the subject of extensive debate and clinical investigation based on two landmark studies in the early 1990s from the Veterans Affairs Laryngeal Cancer Study Group (Wolf, 1991) and the Intergroup Radiation Therapy Oncology Group (RTOG 91-11) (Forastiere et al., 2013). These studies found no difference between the overall survival of patients who received radiation-based treatments with chemotherapy (chemoradiation) and of those who underwent a total laryngectomy. Despite advances in

Box 6-3
Chemotherapy intensifies swallowing toxicity (adverse effects on swallowing function). Patients who undergo chemotherapy as part of their treatment regimen have reported more difficulty swallowing than patients who undergo single-modality treatment (Burnip, Owen, Barker, & Patterson, 2013; Fung et al., 2005; Guadagnolo et al., 2005; Hutcheson et al., 2008; LoTempio et al., 2005). As an example, Burnip et al. (2013) examined three measures of swallowing in a cohort of 123 patients with advanced LC at least 12 months after treatment with laryngectomy and adjuvant radiation therapy, radiotherapy alone, or concurrent chemoradiation. The majority of these patients had some difficulty swallowing, and less than 45% of the participants in the chemoradiation group could manage a normal diet.

methods of radiation delivery and improvements in chemotherapy, the overall survival rate after the use of these treatments has not changed over the years (Rosenthal et al., 2015).

Impact of Treatment Choices on Swallowing

It is well documented that preserving the larynx via nonsurgical treatments is not synonymous with functional preservation of the swallow (Forastiere, Weber, & Trotti, 2015; Hutcheson et al., 2008; Laccourreye et al., 2012). Thus, patients cured of their disease may experience devastating consequences for their *health-related quality of life* as a result of adverse effects from these treatments. Specifically, swallowing difficulty 24 months after the completion of treatment was reported by less than 30% of the patients in the Veterans Affairs study (Wolf, 1991) and by 15% in RTOG 91-11 (Forastiere et al., 2003) (Box 6-3). In a post hoc analysis 10 years later, Forastiere et al. (2013) noted a higher rate of non–cancer-related deaths in their chemoradiotherapy group, which the authors postulated was a result of unrecognized late treatment effects such as dysphagia and aspiration with pneumonia (Forastiere et al., 2013).

Communicating the Impact of Treatment Decisions on Swallowing

In presenting treatment options to patients with advanced-stage LC, clinicians should engage in a discussion of the true functional outcome of the organ-preservation approach beyond overall survival. It has been the assumption that total laryngectomy is more devastating to patients. However, a dysfunctional larynx with associated aspiration, and potentially pneumonia, may result in a greater negative impact on health-related quality of life.

Additional considerations when presenting treatment options to patients include the patient's functional status and age:

- A patient who presents with a dysfunctional larynx and severe airway compromise at diagnosis is likely to remain as such after treatment and, thus, would be a poor candidate for an organ-preservation approach (Forastiere et al., 2015).

- A patient's performance status should be sufficiently robust to endure the acute treatment toxicities of chemoradiotherapy. The patient should also be able to adhere to the daily radiation regime as well as have access to social and supportive care.

- Patient age is also a variable in treatment considerations. Using Surveillance, Epidemiology and End Results (SEER) data from the National Cancer Institute, Gourin et al. (2014) found a survival advantage in elderly patients who underwent surgery followed by radiation therapy over those who were treated with an organ-preservation approach. The data showed an

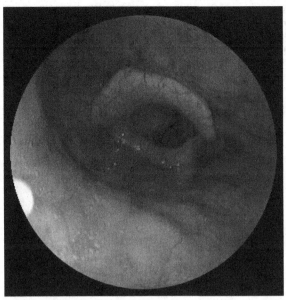

Figure 6-1. Typical view of vocal folds and surrounding structures during FEES. (Reprinted with permission from Med Chaos [own work] [CC BY-SA 3.0 (http://creativecommons.org/licenses/by-sa/3.0)], via Wikimedia Commons at https://commons.wikimedia.org/wiki/File:Normal_Epiglottis.jpg.)

increase in swallowing and airway impairments after chemoradiation therapy with decreased survival as a result of noncancer concerns.

VARIABLES IN THE ASSESSMENT OF SWALLOWING OUTCOMES

Most studies that reported swallowing outcomes after chemoradiation therapy for advanced head and neck cancers were heterogeneous in their participant profiles with respect to the site of disease. Only a few reports of outcomes after an organ-preservation approach were focused just on patients with LC (Burnip et al., 2013; Dworkin et al., 2006; Fung et al., 2005; Guadagnolo et al., 2005; Hutcheson et al., 2008; Stenson et al., 2012). Most studies have included patients with a variety of lesion sites in the head and neck.

Complicating the situation further, multiple methods are used to evaluate swallowing outcomes in patients with LC. Patient-reported outcomes of swallow function, such as the M.D. Anderson Dysphagia Inventory (Chen et al., 2001), contain patient-completed disease-specific emotional, physical, or functional outcomes after treatment. Other studies use instrumental procedures such as the *Videofluoroscopic Swallow Study* (VFSS) or *Fiberoptic Endoscopic Evaluation of Swallow* (FEES), which provide a detailed record of swallowing physiology via imaging (Figures 6-1 and 6-2; Box 6-4), whereas other studies use clinician-administered rating scales that link swallow severity and diet tolerance. Other studies examine specific patient factors to draw conclusions about swallow competency, such as whether the patient depends on a G-tube or tracheotomy, uses nutritional supplements, is experiencing weight loss, has a history of pneumonia, or is on a modified diet (Hutcheson et al., 2008). Yet, the absence of any of the previously mentioned factors (i.e., lack of need for nutritional supplements, no history of pneumonia) may not indicate that a patient truly has normal swallowing physiology. The variability in study methodologies makes it difficult to draw conclusions about functional outcomes related to swallowing in patients with LC. The next sections present known information relative to swallow function after the possible treatments for LC.

Figure 6-2. Lateral view of oral, head, and laryngeal structures on radiographic image from a VFSS. (Reprinted with permission from Normaler Schluck-00.jpg (and others): Hellerhoff derivative work: Anka Friedrich [CC BY-SA 3.0 (http://creativecommons.org/licenses/by-sa/3.0)], via Wikimedia Commons at https://commons.wikimedia.org/wiki/File%3ANormal_barium_swallow_animation.gif.)

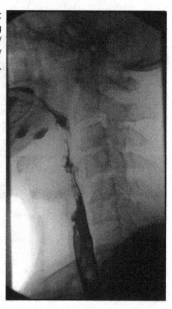

Box 6-4

The two major imaging methods used to assess swallowing include the FEES and the VFSS.

1. FEES: Sometimes referred to as *endoscopic evaluation* of swallowing, FEES involves the insertion of a flexible nasoendoscope, connected to a camera and computer monitor, into the nasal cavity. Once inserted, the scope is then guided below the soft palate and positioned in the superior pharynx. Once positioned appropriately, various consistencies of solids and liquids, mixed with food coloring, are swallowed by the patient. The movement of these materials through the pharynx is then monitored on the computer screen. After the swallow the scope is advanced to just above the vocal folds to look for evidence of laryngeal penetration or aspiration. Proper airway protection at and above the level of the vocal folds can be assessed. Structural and functional issues of the larynx, pharynx, and palate can also be assessed via this assessment measure, and pooling of secretions in the pharynx or larynx can also be viewed. (See Figure 6-1 for the visualization provided by this assessment method.)

   ○ Advantages of FEES

     • May be performed on patients in a variety of positions and locations (e.g., the bedside)

     • Relatively inexpensive

     • Can be performed without food or liquid (i.e., saliva swallows may be viewed) if necessary to decrease risk of aspiration

   ○ Disadvantages of FEES

     • Cannot be used to assess oral or esophageal phases of the swallow

     • Aspiration can be inferred but not visualized during the swallow

(continued)

Box 6-4 (CONTINUED)

2. VFSS: Sometimes referred to as videofluoroscopy, a *modified barium swallow* (MBS), or cookie swallow, the VFSS takes place in the radiology department and involves the patient ingesting various liquids and solids coated with barium. During each swallow, swallowing anatomy (oral cavity, oropharynx and laryngopharynx, and esophagus) and physiology are recorded using radiographic imaging. The VFSS provides comprehensive information about how efficiently and effectively a food bolus moves through the oral cavity and pharynx and into the esophagus, and whether aspiration and/or penetration has taken place. (See Figure 6-2 for the visualization provided by this assessment method.)

  ○ Advantages of the VFSS

   • Assesses all phases of the swallow effectively and provides information about the etiology of aspiration and/or penetration and bolus-transit problems

   • Can be used to assess the swallow via a side or front view of the head, neck, and esophagus

   • Can provide information about esophageal function and deficits

  ○ Disadvantages of the VFSS

   • Cannot be performed at the bedside; must take place in a radiology suite with the patient positioned upright

   • Exposes the patient to radiation and requires costly radiology equipment and personnel

Content adapted from Marcotte's (2006), *Critical Review: Effectiveness of FEES in comparison to VFSS at identifying aspiration.* Retrieved from https://www.uwo.ca/fhs/csd/ebp/reviews/2006-07/Marcotte.pdf.

The following resources provide additional information about these assessment tools:

• http://www.asha.org/public/speech/swallowing/Videofluoroscopic-Swallowing-Study/

• http://www.asha.org/public/speech/swallowing/endoscopy/

SWALLOW FUNCTION AFTER RADIATION-BASED TREATMENT

Dysphagia in patients with LC treated with radiation with or without chemotherapy is commonplace and can affect swallow safety (aspiration) and efficiency (residue). Swallow function after radiotherapy alone for early LC is usually preserved once the acute effects of radiotherapy such as pain, *dysgeusia* (persistently abnormal taste in the mouth), and edema have dissipated (Smith et al., 2003). These patients suffer more from dysphonia than dysphagia in the immediate posttreatment period and, over time, usually resume a normal diet of solids and liquids.

Locally advanced cancers of the larynx (stages T3 and T4) portend higher rates of dysphagia irrespective of the disease subsite. In a large study devoted only to patients with advanced LC treated with an organ-preservation approach, Hutcheson et al. (2008) found that 84% of the patients aspirated and 44% did so silently on VFSS after treatment. These toxicities were observed to be more significant in elderly patients. Examining Surveillance, Epidemiology and End Results data,

Gourin et al. (2014) found an increased incidence of dysphagia, weight loss, esophageal stricture, airway obstruction, and pneumonia in elderly patients 1 year after treatment.

Radiation toxicities occur for most patients during their treatment and are intensified with accelerated radiation therapy schedules, especially with concurrent chemotherapy. After 1 or 2 weeks, treatment induces inflammation of the radiation site and causes the following symptoms:

- *Erythema* (redness)
- *Mucositis* (inflammation of mucous membranes)
- *Necrosis* (cell/tissue death)
- *Sloughing* (shedding of dead tissue)

In addition, patients may experience severe dysphonia, dysphagia with aspiration, and odyno-phagia (painful swallowing) during treatment. G-tubes may be placed to mitigate the pain caused by oral intake.

In general, the acute inflammatory changes that result from treatment resolve over the first few months after treatment is completed. However, long-term radiation effects result in damage to the DNA and causes hyperactivation of the protein transforming growth factor beta (TGF-β), which in turn activates cellular pathways to induce fibrosis (thickening of connective tissue) (Johns et al., 2012). Fibrotic collagen deposits reduce tissue compliance and ultimately restrict movement of laryngeal, tongue-base, pharyngeal, and hyolaryngeal musculature.

Radiation-induced fibrosis may result in compromised airway protection and, hence, dysphagia. In particular, laryngeal muscles that adduct the vocal folds and aryepiglottic muscles that facilitate epiglottic inversion may be affected secondarily by the acute radiation-induced inflammatory response (Johns et al., 2012). Vocal folds may stiffen and adduct incompletely, which increases the risk for aspiration during the swallow. The arytenoid cartilages can also become fibrotic, edema-tous, and sluggish in movement. Weakening of the epiglottis after radiation therapy is common, and in some cases, severe scarring obliterates it completely. Intensity-modulated radiation therapy has been associated with stricture formation in some patients with LC, especially when their oral structures are affected by radiation (Box 6-5). Weak base-of-tongue retraction that leads to incomplete contact with the posterior pharyngeal wall during swallowing may also cause an accumulation of residue in the pharyngeal recesses that can be aspirated after a swallow (Wall et al., 2013).

Fibrosis may occur within only a few months after treatment is completed. At other times, radiation fibrosis occurs gradually without the patient being aware until swallow safety has become compromised significantly. Specifically, chronic dysphagia and silent aspiration may, in some cases, become problematic approximately 5 or more years after radiation treatment has been completed. With such severe late-stage effects, the only viable alternative for the patient to continue eating orally may be laryngectomy.

The concept of the new normal bears mentioning as a patient learns to develop functional coping strategies for an insidiously developing problem. Patients may unconsciously alter their diet to include more moist or cohesive items or prefer to drink thicker beverages reducing coughing. It may seem second nature to the patient (and their family members) to cough, expectorate, and clear the throat frequently during meals. The new normal obscures the relationship between patient perceptions of dysphagia and physiologic findings in which patients underestimate the difficulty they experience with eating or drinking (Logemann, 1998).

Swallow Function After Surgery

There are many surgeries that can be offered to patients with LC. The size and location of the laryngeal tumor will dictate what is possible, but other variables need to be considered, including vocal fold mobility, age, comorbidities, and social and cognitive issues. Institutions may favor certain resections on the basis of philosophy and the expertise of their team. The speech-language

---

BOX 6-5

Intensity-modulated radiation therapy is an advanced radiotherapy that may reduce the exposure of healthy tissue to radiation by targeting photon beams to the shape of a circumscribed tumor.

The following resource might be helpful for obtaining additional information regarding intensity-modulated radiation therapy: http://www.mayoclinic.org/tests-procedures/imrt/basics/definition/prc-20013330

---

pathologist (SLP) plays a role in treatment decisions in the determination of baseline laryngeal function, because pretreatment voice and swallow function can predict postsurgical outcomes (Patterson & Wilson, 2011). In general, larger resections predict more significant changes in swallow function.

Minimally Invasive Surgical Procedures

With small stage T1 or T2 laryngeal tumors, minimally invasive endoscopic surgery for resecting the lesion may be appropriate. Surgery can be done with a traditional cold-steel technique (surgery in which unheated cutting instruments are used) or with carbon dioxide laser microsurgery. Many patients are able to initiate oral intake of food/drink without appreciable dysphagia immediately after surgery, whereas others have transient dysphagia. In general, patients who undergo these minimally invasive procedures are expected to return to normal swallow function (O'Hara et al., 2016; Suárez et al., 2012). No adjuvant treatment is recommended after these surgeries.

Partial Laryngectomy

Partial removal of the larynx is performed for oncologic management with the goal of maintaining voice and swallow function (Ogura, Marks, & Freeman, 1980). There are several varieties of partial laryngectomy (described later in this chapter). However, it is important to understand that in all partial laryngectomy surgeries, airway protection is compromised to some degree, and the risk for aspiration is high (Rademaker et al., 1993). In addition to laryngeal resection, patients may also require postoperative radiation, which may further threaten their laryngeal function (Laccourreye et al., 2000).

Careful selection of patients for partial laryngectomy is important. Their pulmonary status and frailty must be examined, because postoperative aspiration of secretions and chronic microaspiration of liquids is often unavoidable (Sasaki, Leder, Acton, & Maune, 2006). Patients need to complete an extensive course of swallow therapy and undergo training in compensatory strategies. Using these strategies can be challenging; therefore, the cognitive status of the patient and his or her motivation for rehabilitation should be evaluated as well. It is important to share with patients that, although partial laryngectomy can be successful initially, swallow function may deteriorate with time as a result of age-related changes and late radiation effects. As a result, patients may ultimately require additional surgery (i.e., total laryngectomy) to eliminate chronic aspiration (Bagwell, Leder, & Sasaki, 2015).

Supraglottic Laryngectomy

Supraglottic laryngectomy is a horizontal superior resection of the larynx above the true vocal folds, and it can be performed as an open or endoscopic surgery. Therefore, the true vocal folds remain, but the false vocal folds, aryepiglottic folds, epiglottis, and superior thyroid cartilage are resected, with or without the hyoid bone (Hirano, Kurita, Tateishi, & Matsuoka, 1987). Infrahyoid muscles are detached and the superior laryngeal nerve may be damaged, affecting sensation and the glottic closure reflex during the swallow. In the endoscopic laser approach, resection of the hyoid bone and thyroid cartilage are spared, and the laryngeal nerve sectioning is avoided, which therefore may preserve the glottal closure reflex (Sasaki et al., 2006). Swallow function after supraglottic laryngectomy is characterized by aspiration during and after the swallow because of decreased laryngeal closure. If there is tumor invasion into the base of the tongue, extended supraglottic laryngectomy is necessary, which means more resection and potentially more significant dysphagia characterized by weak bolus propulsion and *pharyngeal stasis* (residue in the pharyngeal cavity during swallowing) (Rademaker et al., 1993).

Hemilaryngectomy

Hemilaryngectomy is also a partial laryngectomy, but in contrast to the horizontal resection done with supraglottic laryngectomy, it is a vertical resection. The classic surgery involves the division of thyroid cartilage medially and includes unilateral false and true vocal folds. A pedicled muscle flap can be used to rebuild the defect and improve glottic closure (Amin & Koufman, 2001). Frontolateral laryngectomy is a variation that includes the anterior commissure and one-third of the healthy vocal fold, or resection can extend posteriorly to include the arytenoid. The hemilaryngectomy must be performed as an open surgery, and it requires a temporary postoperative tracheostomy. Swallow function will be characterized initially by aspiration because of incomplete laryngeal closure, but it usually recovers faster than it would after other types of partial laryngectomy (Rademaker et al., 1993).

Supracricoid Laryngectomy

A final partial laryngectomy is the *supracricoid laryngectomy*, which has evolved to be known as the cricohyoidopexy (CHP) or cricohyoidoepiglottopexy (CHEP). Resection is horizontal and includes the entire thyroid cartilage, true vocal folds, and paralaryngeal spaces; the cricoid cartilage and at least one arytenoid are preserved. The hyoid bone remains, and the cricoid cartilage is sutured to the hyoid bone for better airway protection. In CHP, the epiglottis is spared, but in CHEP, the epiglottis is resected (Bron, Brossard, Monnier, & Pasche, 2000). Functional results after CHP should be more favorable than those after CHEP, because the presence of the partial epiglottis aids airway protection (Holsinger, Laccourreye, Weinstein, Diaz, & McWhorter, 2005). The expected dysphagia is significant and characterized by aspiration caused by neoglottis incompetence (inability of surgically reshaped physiology to protect the airway) and impaired movement of both the base of the tongue and the larynx. However, Lewin et al. (2008) reported that 81% of the patients in their study were ultimately able to return to oral intake after supracricoid laryngectomy.

Total Laryngectomy and Total Laryngopharyngectomy

The entire larynx, including all cartilages, intrinsic muscles, hyoid bone, epiglottis, and upper tracheal rings are resected in a total laryngectomy. The trachea is then brought out through the front of the neck, and a permanent stoma is created for breathing. Total laryngectomy may be used as the initial treatment for large stage T3 or T4 laryngeal tumors or as salvage resection for recurrent disease after primary radiation (Stoeckli, Pawlik, & Lipp, 2000). If tumor invades the pharyngeal walls, a pharyngectomy may be performed also, and then a radial forearm flap will be used for the construction of a neopharynx (Scharpf & Esclamado, 2003; Withrow et al., 2007).

The characteristics of dysphagia after total laryngectomy differ from those after partial laryngectomy. Because there is complete separation between the trachea and esophagus, aspiration is not possible after total laryngectomy. However, the changes in anatomy and physiology result in a weaker swallow. Normally, when the larynx rises, it pulls open the cricopharyngeus, which allows the food bolus to enter the cervical esophagus. Therefore, when the larynx has been removed, bolus movement must be driven via tongue propulsion and pharyngeal wall contraction, and sometimes these forces are diminished from previous radiation or resection (Maclean, Cotton, & Perry, 2009). Therefore, the swallow is weaker, and pharyngeal stasis with food and liquid often occurs (Balfe, 1990). To help with this issue, many surgeons routinely perform *myotomy* (a procedure in which muscle fibers are cut) of the cricopharyngeus at the time of surgery to improve clearance of the bolus through the neopharynx to the cervical esophagus (Ward, Bishop, Frisby, & Stevens, 2002).

The prevalence of dysphagia after total laryngectomy is unknown, but it is estimated that 17% to 70% of patients will have some form of dysphagia after their laryngectomy (Maclean et al., 2009). Because of a weaker swallow after total laryngectomy, many patients do best functionally with a soft diet and using multiple swallows and a liquid wash to clear residue. However, some patients are restricted to liquids because of a weak swallow and may require nutritional supplements for weight maintenance. Oral intake may also decrease as a result of diminished senses of smell and taste, owing to a lack of airflow to the nose and mouth (Maclean et al., 2009).

The following is a list of additional issues that might affect swallowing after laryngectomy:

- *Pharyngocutaneous fistulas*, connections between the pharynx and cervical skin around the surgical incision, reported at an incidence of 26.3% (Timmermans et al., 2014), can develop during healing and may delay the initiation of oral intake. Previous chemoradiation is a risk factor for fistula development. Patients usually just need more time to heal and may require NPO (*nil per os*) and G-tube use for an extended period.

- *Anastomosis stricture*, the development of scar tissue at the junction of the neopharynx and cervical esophagus, causes a narrowed esophageal opening and may result in dysphagia (Sweeny et al., 2012). *Esophageal dilation*, a procedure that stretches a narrowed area of the esophagus can provide relief, and this procedure may be needed once, serially, or periodically for a lifetime to maintain swallow function (Scharpf & Esclamado, 2003).

- Some patients after total laryngectomy are found to have a *pseudoepiglottis*, which is a structure near the base of the tongue that arises from a vertical or T-shaped closure technique that resembles an epiglottis (Davis, Vincent, Sharpshay, & Strong, 1982). Food and liquid can pool in the fold and cause more significant pharyngeal residue.

Because the vocal folds are removed in total laryngectomy, patients who undergo this surgery must find and use new methods of communication. Their options include using an electrolarynx, esophageal speech, or tracheoesophageal speech, which is the most popular choice. These modes of communication are described in more depth in Chapter 5. Regarding swallowing, it is important to note that when a tracheoesophageal voice prosthesis is in place, aspiration is possible if there is leakage through or around the prosthesis. A clinician should be able to visualize and differentiate leakage through or around the prosthesis by having the patient drink liquid (something with a visible color [e.g., milk, grape juice]) and then observe an anterior view of the prosthesis through the stoma. Leakage is typically also visible with videofluoroscopic imaging. It may be caused by Candida obstructing closure of prosthesis's valve (Busscher, Geertsema-Doornbusch, & van der Mei, 1997). In these cases, leakage is resolved when the voice prosthesis is replaced. Leakage around the prosthesis indicates an overdilated tracheoesophageal tract (Hutcheson, Lewin, Sturgis, & Risser, 2011), which can be complex to manage. If leakage through or around the voice prosthesis cannot be resolved, aspiration will persist, and the patient will be at risk for aspiration pneumonia.

EVALUATION

Regardless of staging and treatment choices, it is the SLP who is challenged with evaluating and treating swallow dysfunction across the continuum. Any discussion of swallow function after treatment for LC requires a two-pronged analysis, including that of the physiologic changes over time and patient-reported outcome with respect to swallow function. It is not uncommon for patients to under-report their dysphagia; thus, dissonance often exists between physiologic findings on instrumental evaluations of swallowing and patient perceptions (Patterson & Wilson, 2011).

Changes in swallow function throughout the continuum of a patient's disease and careful selection of time points for evaluating swallow outcomes are critical for depicting the true picture of a patient's swallow function. Baseline assessment provides an important marker against which to measure posttreatment function. Many patients with stage T1 or T2 LC present with no swallow problems at the baseline evaluation. However, patients with stage T3 or T4 disease, along with vocal fold immobility and bulky extralaryngeal lesions that affect closure of the laryngeal vestibule, may have severe difficulty swallowing, and in some cases, a tracheotomy may be required to support their respiration (Stenson et al., 2012).

If a patient undergoes resection, postoperative evaluation is essential before starting oral intake, particularly after partial laryngectomy, and it should take place shortly after surgery when deemed appropriate by the surgeon. In patients with LC treated with primary radiation or chemoradiation, baseline swallow should be determined, and then function should be monitored throughout treatment for acute changes in swallow function. Finally, swallow function may need to be evaluated years after treatment because of late effects of treatment or changes that result from comorbidities and aging.

Evaluation should start with a clinical evaluation, often termed the *Bedside Swallow Evaluation* (BSE). The process of a BSE is as follows:

1. The SLP completes a thorough chart review to understand the patient's medical history, treatment, extent of resection, etc.

2. Oral-motor function is assessed to determine cranial nerve function, which may provide insight into the patient's expected swallow function.

3. Cognition and respiratory status are then considered to determine the patient's readiness for trials of food and liquid.

4. If deemed appropriate, the SLP then begins trials with materials of different consistencies and observes the patient swallowing.

5. A judgment is made about swallow function on the basis of signs of aspiration, timeliness of mastication and swallow, laryngeal rise, and signs of pharyngeal residue.

A BSE is noninvasive, in that no instrumentation is used to visualize a patient's swallow function internally. For some patients, this sort of evaluation is adequate; however, because the incidence of silent aspiration is high in patients treated surgically or with chemoradiation, an instrumental evaluation might be necessary. Readily available options for instrumental examination are VFSS and FEES (see Box 6-4 for additional details). Visualization is necessary to understand the nature of the swallow dysfunction and to plan treatment. VFSS provides lateral and anterior-posterior radiographic views of the physiology of the neck to show the recreated anatomy and/or postradiation changes. VFSS yields important information about the following conditions:

- Oral, pharyngeal, and esophageal phases of the swallow (Table 6-1)
- Velopharyngeal closure
- Base-of-tongue retraction
- Laryngeal elevation and closure
- Aspiration
- Pharyngeal residue
- Cricopharyngeal opening

FEES uses a flexible nasoendoscope to provide a direct view of the pharyngeal anatomy so that resection and reconstruction can be visualized. Postradiation changes (e.g., blunted epiglottis or fibrotic tissue) are also recognizable. Glottic closure and secretion management can be observed before presenting any food or liquid. Only the pharyngeal phase of a patient's swallow function can be viewed with FEES, but this type of diagnostic study can identify velopharyngeal insufficiency, aspiration, and pharyngeal residue.

With any instrumental evaluation, trials with different bolus consistencies should be run to determine if a patient is able to swallow certain thicknesses of liquids/foods more safely than

TABLE 6-1		
STAGES OF A NORMAL SWALLOW		
SWALLOWING STAGE	CHARACTERISTICS OF STAGE	DYSPHAGIA SYMPTOMS
Oral	1. Patient introduces food into mouth 2. Food mixes with saliva to soften it and form a bolus 3. The tongue pushes the bolus to the back of the mouth in preparation for the pharyngeal stage of swallowing	• Difficulty closing lips around a spoon or fork to form a labial seal • Difficulty with the process of chewing or forming a bolus • Inability to move bolus to the back of the mouth

Pharyngeal	1. As the bolus moves out of the mouth and into the pharynx, the vocal folds close to protect the trachea
	2. The larynx rises in the throat and the epiglottis covers the trachea to keep the bolus from entering the airway
		• Aspiration can occur if a bolus touches the vocal folds or enters the lungs; specific symptoms of aspiration include the following:
		  ○ Coughing during or after eating
		  ○ Gagging on food when trying to swallow
		  ○ A choking sensation when swallowing
		  ○ A wet, gurgly vocal quality after eating
		  ○ Repeated pneumonia or fever

Esophageal	1. The bolus leaves the pharynx and enters the esophagus, where muscles squeeze the bolus to move it into the stomach	• Heartburn • Vomiting • Burping • Abdominal pain
		Logemann, 1998

others. Patients who have undergone a partial laryngectomy will often be at greater risk for aspirating thin liquids, and thicker consistencies will likely be tolerated better initially because they travel more slowly and are easier for a patient to control.

INTERVENTION FOR IMPROVING SWALLOW FUNCTION

The management of patients with LC continues from diagnosis to beyond completion of treatment, and regular and frequent contact is appropriate, particularly during chemoradiation therapy. The following recommendations should be considered during this time:

- The patient should continue to swallow to maintain muscular action and to reduce the potential formation of fibrosis.

- The patient should complete SLP-provided prophylactic swallow exercises that focus on volitional and exaggerated airway protection during swallowing to prevent aspiration (Hutcheson et al., 2013). To increase adherence, the exercises should be realistic, targeted at impairment, and be understood by and important to the patient.

- For patients with submental lymphedema (swelling beneath the chin), consider referral to a specially trained lymphedema therapist, who can assist in reducing the sensation of throat tightness and increase the sensation of bolus flow through the pharynx and cervical esophagus (Lewin et al., 2008).

After evaluation is completed, a course of swallow therapy may be needed. Particularly after partial laryngectomy, an extended course of rehabilitation should be expected. Instrumental evaluation will determine safe consistencies and compensations, and, as previously noted, thicker consistencies usually are tolerated best, at least initially.

In terms of providing strategies for supporting patients in rehabilitating their swallowing function, the following are several compensations and postures (based on type of resection and mechanics of the swallow) to consider:

- The supraglottic swallow and the super-supraglottic swallow employ volitional airway closure before the swallow (Ohmae, 1996).

  o In the supraglottic swallow maneuver, patients are instructed to hold their breath at the level of the glottis, swallow, then cough immediately after the swallow to expel any material in the laryngeal vestibule. Then, they are instructed to swallow once more to clear pharyngeal residue.

  o The super-supraglottic swallow involves the same sequence but with a more effortful breath-hold and more effortful swallow.

- After hemilaryngectomy, a head turn toward the resected side will close off the unilateral pharynx, improve airway closure by placing extrinsic pressure on thyroid cartilage, and direct bolus flow down the opposite side (Logemann, 1998).

- The use of a chin tuck may also be helpful after hemilaryngectomy, because it will push the epiglottis posteriorly and improve airway protection (Welch, 1993).

As an example of how these techniques might be applied, after a supraglottic laryngectomy, swallow therapy may start with trials of purée to practice the supraglottic swallow. Swallow exercises may also be included in therapy to improve laryngeal rise, base-of-tongue retraction, and pharyngeal constriction.

In many cases, the SLP may facilitate rehabilitation of a patient's swallowing mechanism while he or she is receiving alternative means of nutrition (i.e., tube feedings) placed by a gastroenterologist or other medical professional. Alternative nutrition may be necessary if a patient's swallow is deemed unsafe and results in him or her being placed on NPO status. Even when food can be taken by mouth, supplemental nutrition may be necessary. For example, poor appetite or difficulty or pain with chewing or swallowing because of tumor location or side effects from radiation or chemotherapy can result in decreased caloric intake that necessitates tube feedings for supplemental nutrition. In other cases, dietary restrictions to specific consistencies (i.e., pureed foods only) might be prescribed to minimize aspiration risk but might also result in the patient requiring additional nutrition through supplementation, particularly if the patient finds the prescribed consistency less palatable. It is important to note that the collaboration between dietitians and SLPs is imperative in any of these situations to preserve adequate nutrition and facilitate swallowing safety and rehabilitation concurrently in patients with LC.

Box 6-6

The Feeding Tube Awareness Association identifies two main types of feeding tubes: nasogastric and gastric feeding tubes.

1. *Nasogastric* (NG) *feeding tubes* are placed nonsurgically and are intended to provide temporary (up to 3 weeks before placing a new tube) access to nutrition for patients. The NG tube enters the body through the nose and runs down through the nasal cavity to the stomach via the esophagus.

2. Gastric (G)-tubes are placed surgically though the abdominal wall into the stomach and are intended to meet long-term nutritional needs when a patient's oral and pharyngeal structures cannot support a safe and healthy swallow.

The following resource might be helpful for obtaining additional information regarding different types of feeding tubes: https://globalgenes.org/raredaily/types-of-feeding-tubes-and-terms-to-know-by-the-feeding-tube-awareness-foundation/.

The length of swallow rehabilitation varies depending on the extent of resection, the need for postoperative radiation, and patient compliance and motivation. Some patients will need a short-term NG feeding tube, whereas others will require a G-tube while they work toward full oral intake (Wasserman et al., 2001) (Box 6-6).

Rehabilitation is expected to be lengthy as a result of loss of the true and false vocal folds, particularly after supracricoid laryngectomy. Return to oral intake after supracricoid laryngectomy was documented to be at a median of 9.4 weeks in one sample (Lewin et al., 2008). Because of the length of time that patients must refrain from oral feeding, a G-tube is often necessary for those who have undergone supracricoid laryngectomy. Consider Case Studies 6-1 and 6-2 as examples of how treatment for impaired swallow function can vary from one patient to another.

PATIENT-REPORTED OUTCOMES

Adherence to swallow treatment recommendations increase when there is synergy between clinician and patient assessments of function. Thus, it is critical to ascertain patients' feelings toward their swallowing function and any effects that swallowing may have on their overall quality of life. To this end, it is instructive to have patients complete outcome questionnaires that reflect the impact of their swallowing function on their overall quality of life. The M.D. Anderson Dysphagia Inventory (2001) is a widely used, short, and simple-to-complete questionnaire that has been validated with patients with head and neck cancer. Govender et al. (2012) developed and validated the Swallowing Outcome After Laryngectomy (SOAL), a patient-completed questionnaire, the goal of which is to identify patients with dysphagia who may be overlooked or under-reported. Review of questionnaire responses by both the SLP and patient together may help them prioritize and collaborate on treatment goals while also enhancing patient adherence to treatment recommendations. Overall, patients depend on their SLP to help them maintain oral intake of liquids and foods, which directly affects their quality of life.

CONCLUSION

Challenges to swallowing and nutrition are common in patients with LC. The assessment and management of these challenges require a strong understanding of the disease and how its

---

CASE STUDY 6-1

PATIENT NAME: BOB

Clinical Status: newly diagnosed with dysphagia after supraglottic laryngectomy

Bob is a 72-year-old man found to have a supraglottic tumor (stage T2, N1, M0). Because of the location and size of the tumor, he was judged to be a perfect candidate for supraglottic laryngectomy. He seemed to be in good general health, and although he was widowed, he had supportive adult children who were involved in his care. As part of his treatment, Bob planned for postoperative radiation therapy. He underwent the surgery and had a G-tube placed prophylactically because of the expected swallow rehabilitation and planned radiation.

After surgery, Bob underwent a VFSS, which revealed aspiration during his swallow caused by decreased laryngeal closure. He initiated swallow therapy and was trained on the super-supraglottic swallow. It was difficult for him to learn the super-supraglottic swallow; he could demonstrate the compensatory strategy at swallow therapy sessions with SLP guidance, but his children reported that when he went home, he would not remember to do it. Several weeks later, he initiated radiation therapy. The radiation treatment caused quite a few adverse effects; therefore, his swallow therapy was put on hold. After radiation was completed, swallow therapy resumed, but Bob could not master independent performance of the super-supraglottic swallow.

As the SLP got to know Bob well, it became apparent that Bob had cognitive and memory deficits that affected his ability to learn new things. Bob was diagnosed with pneumonia several times while attempting oral intake over the next year. A decision eventually had to be made, because Bob could no longer swallow foods or liquids safely. His treatment team gave Bob two options: total laryngectomy to prevent further pneumonia or removal of all oral feedings, with only the G-tube used to attain all nutrition. His children felt total laryngectomy would be too difficult of an adjustment for him, and they declined this option. Bob continues to be NPO with full tube feedings.

CASE STUDY 6-2

PATIENT NAME: MAGGIE

Clinical Status: 8 years after diagnosis with recurrent dysphagia

Maggie is a 62-year-old woman who presented 8 years ago with a well-differentiated stage T3 squamous cell carcinoma of the left aryepiglottic fold extending into the epiglottis without vallecula, tongue base, or vocal fold involvement. The patient declined surgery in favor of an organ-preservation approach. She was treated with weekly chemotherapy and daily radiation therapy. The patient's course of treatment was complicated by a high-grade cervical esophageal stricture that was diagnosed immediately after her treatment was completed. She underwent a cervical esophageal dilation, and her G-tube was removed 6 months after treatment was completed. Besides xerostomia, which necessitated a liquid wash, the patient resumed a regular diet, including meats and bread, and she was able to take small pills. She was not aware of aspirating and did not feel any food getting caught in her throat. She quit smoking but developed mild symptoms of chronic obstructive pulmonary disease (COPD), which required bronchodilators for treatment of the condition.

(continued)

CASE STUDY 6-2 (CONTINUED)

A VFSS was performed 4 years after her treatment because Maggie and her SLP noted increasing oral secretions. This evaluation revealed trace silent laryngeal penetration and aspiration of thin liquids during the swallow as a result of sluggish closure of the laryngeal vestibule in the context of full hyolaryngeal elevation and anterior movement. To compensate for this problem, Maggie was shown how to use a head turn to the left together with a chin-tuck posture when swallowing, which was beneficial for her. The super-supraglottic swallow maneuver also increased her airway protection.

Maggie underwent a course of swallow therapy, during which she learned and appeared to habituate the strategies she was shown. She continued on a regular diet. One year later, she returned for a re-evaluation after two episodes of aspiration pneumonia, the last of which required intubation and hospitalization. Instrumental re-evaluation with a VFSS revealed weak tongue-base retraction, impaired hyolaryngeal elevation, and delayed and incomplete closure of the laryngeal vestibule, which were resulting in frank but silent aspiration of thin liquids after the swallow. Thicker consistencies were evaluated as being safer for Maggie, but they were associated with increased residue.

Maggie declined placement of a G-tube. She was relieved that the swallow strategies she had forgotten were still effective in eradicating her aspiration, and she was willing to alter her diet to include more uniform textures, use the super-supraglottic swallow technique, and return for regular swallow treatment to reinforce these therapeutic strategies. In addition, Maggie was referred to a respiratory therapist in light of her worsening COPD. Maggie developed and established her new normal swallow behavior but remains at risk for pneumonia and aspiration/dysphagia-related complications.

---

treatments may affect the anatomy and physiology of swallowing and airway protection. Because both the treatments for LC and the primary disease typically compromise swallowing function, dysphagia may be a primary consideration from the time of diagnosis to well after the conclusion of LC treatment. An SLP with specialized experience in working with patients with LC is essential for assessing swallow safety throughout the continuum of care, educating patients about the impact of LC and its management on the anatomy and physiology of their swallowing mechanism, advocating for patient safety through diet modifications and swallowing maneuvers, and facilitating exercises to rehabilitate swallow function. In the case that oral intake is inadequate because of the effects of laryngeal tumors or radiation or cannot be maintained because of swallowing concerns, collaboration between the SLP and a dietitian is vitally important for monitoring and preserving nutritional intake and swallowing safety from diagnosis to after treatment.

REFERENCES

Amin, M. R., & Koufman, J. A. (2001). Hemicricoidectomy for voice rehabilitation following hemilaryngectomy with ipsilateral arytenoid removal. *Annals of Otolaryngology, Rhinology, and Laryngology, 110*, 514–518.

Bagwell, K., Leder, S. B., & Sasaki, C. T. (2015). Is partial laryngectomy safe forever? *American Journal of Otolaryngology, 36*, 437–441.

Balfe, D. M. (1990). Dysphagia after laryngeal surgery: Radiologic assessment. *Dysphagia, 5*, 20–34.

Bron, L., Brossard, E., Monnier, P., & Pasche, P. (2000). Supracricoid partial laryngectomy with cricohyoidoepiglottopexy and cricohyoidopexy for glottic and supraglottic carcinomas. *The Laryngoscope, 110*, 627–634.

Burnip, E., Owen, S. J., Barker, S., & Patterson, J. M. (2013). Swallowing outcomes following surgical and nonsurgical treatment for advanced laryngeal cancer. *Journal of Laryngology and Otology, 127*, 1116–1121.

Busscher, H. J., Geertsema-Doornbusch, G. I., & van der Mei, H. C. (1997). Adhesion to silicone rubber of yeasts and bacteria isolated from voice prostheses: Influence of salivary conditioning films. *Journal of Biomedical Materials Research, 34*, 201–209.

Chen, A. Y., Frankowski, R., Bishop-Leone, J., Hebert, T., Leyk, S., Lewin, J., & Goepfert, H. (2001). The development and validation of a dysphagia-specific quality-of-life questionnaire for patients with head and neck cancer: The M. D. anderson dysphagia inventory. *Archives of Otolaryngology–Head & Neck Surgery, 127*(7), 870–876.

Davis, R. K., Vincent, M. E., Sharpshay, S. M., & Strong, M. S. (1982). The anatomy and complications of "T" versus vertical closure of the hypopharynx after laryngectomy. *The Laryngoscope, 92*, 16–22.

Dworkin, J. P., Hill, S. L., Stachler, R. J., Meleca, R. J., & Kewson, D. (2006). Swallowing function outcomes following nonsurgical therapy for advanced-stage laryngeal carcinoma. *Dysphagia, 21*(1), 66–74. doi:10.1007/s00455-005-9001-8

Forastiere, A. A., Goepfert, H., Maor, M., Pajak, T., Morrison, W., Glisson, B., … Cooper (2003). Concurrent chemotherapy and radiotherapy for organ preservation in advanced laryngeal cancer. *New England Journal of Medicine, 349*, 2091–2098.

Forastiere, A. A., Weber, R. S., & Trotti, A. (2015). Organ preservation for advanced larynx cancer: Issues and outcomes. *Journal of Clinical Oncology, 33*, 3262–3268.

Forastiere, A. A., Zhang, Q., Weber, R. S., Maor, M. H., Goepfert, H., Pajak, T. F., … Cooper, J. S. (2013). Long-term results of RTOG 91–11: A comparison of three nonsurgical treatment strategies to preserve the larynx in patients with locally advanced larynx cancer. *Journal of Clinical Oncology, 31*, 845–852.

Fung, K., Lyden, T. H., Lee, J., Urba, S. G., Worden, F., Eisbruch, A., … Wolf, G. T. (2005). Voice and swallowing outcomes of an organ-preservation trial for advanced laryngeal cancer. *International Journal of Radiation Oncology, Biology, Physics, 63*, 1395–1399.

Gourin, C. G., Dy, S. M., Herbert, R. J., Blackford, A. L., Quon, H., Forastiere, A. A., . . . Frick, K. D. (2014). Treatment, survival, and costs of laryngeal cancer care in the elderly. *The Laryngoscope, 124*(8), 1827–1835. doi:10.1002/lary.24574

Govender, R., Lee, M. T., Davies, T. C., Twinn, C. E., Katsoulis, K. L., Payten, C. L., . . . Drinnan, M. (2012). Development and preliminary validation of a patient-reported outcome measure for swallowing after total laryngectomy (SOAL questionnaire). *Clinical Otolaryngology : Official Journal of ENT-UK ; Official Journal of Netherlands Society for Oto-Rhino-Laryngology & Cervico-Facial Surgery, 37*(6), 452–459. doi:10.1111/coa.12036

Guadagnolo, B. A., Haddad, R. I., Posner, M. R., Weeks, L., Norris, C. M., Sullivan, C. A., … Tishler, R. (2005). Organ preservation and treatment toxicity with induction chemotherapy followed by radiation therapy or chemoradiation for advanced laryngeal cancer. *American Journal of Clinical Oncology, 28*, 371–378.

Hirano, M., Kurita, S., Tateishi, M., Matsuoka, H. (1987). Deglutition following supraglottic horizontal laryngectomy. *Annals of Otology, Rhinology & Laryngology, 96*, 7–11.

Holsinger, F. C., Laccourreye, O., Weinstein, G. S., Diaz, E. M., & McWhorter, A. J. (2005). Technical refinements in the supracricoid partial laryngectomy to optimize functional outcomes. *Journal of the American College of Surgeons, 201*, 809–820.

Hutcheson, K. A., Barringer, D. A., Rosenthanl, D. I., May, A., H., Roberts, D. B., & Lewin, J. B. (2008). Swallowing outcomes after radiotherapy for laryngeal carcinoma. *Otolaryngology–Head and Neck Surgery, 134*, 178–183.

Hutcheson, K. A., Bhayani, M. K., Beadle, B. M., Gold, K. A., Shinn, E. H., Lai, S. Y., & Lewin, J. (2013). Eat and exercise during radiotherapy or chemoradiotherapy for pharyngeal cancers: Use it or lose it. *JAMA Otolaryngology–Head & Neck Surgery, 139*, 1127–1134.

Hutcheson, K. A., Lewin, J. S., Sturgis, E. M., & Risser, J. (2011). Outcomes and adverse events of enlarged tracheoesophageal puncture after total laryngectomy. *The Laryngoscope, 121*, 1455–1461.

Johns, M. M., Kolachala, V., Berg, E., Muller, S., Creighton, F. X., & Branski, R. C. (2012). Radiation fibrosis of the vocal fold: From man to mouse. *The Laryngoscope, 122*, S107-S125.

Laccourreye, O., Hans, S., Borzog-Grayeli, A., Maulard-Durdux, C., Brasnu, D., & Housset, M. (2000). Complications of postoperative radiation therapy after partial laryngectomy in supraglottic cancer: A long term evaluation. *Otolaryngology–Head Neck Surgery, 122*, 752–757.

Laccourreye, O., Malinvaud, D., Holsinger, F. C., Consoli, S., Menard, M., & Bonfils, P. (2012). Trade-off between survival and laryngeal preservation in advanced laryngeal cancer: The otorhinolaryngology patient's perspective. *Annals of Otology, Rhinology, and Laryngology, 121*, 570–575.

Lewin, J. S., Hutcheson, K. A., Barringer, D. A., May, A. H., Roberts, D. B., Holsinger, F. C., & Diaz Jr., E. M. (2008). Functional analysis of swallowing outcomes after supracricoid partial laryngectomy. *Head & Neck, 30*, 559–566.

Logemann, J. A. (1998). *Evaluation and treatment of swallowing disorders*. Austin, TX: Pro-Ed.

LoTempio, M. M., Wang, K. H., Sadeghi, A., Delacure, M. D., Julliard, G. F., & Wang, M. B. (2005). Comparison of quality of life outcomes in laryngeal cancer patients following chemoradiation vs. total laryngectomy. *Otolaryngology–Head and Neck Surgery, 132*, 948–953.

Maclean, J., Cotton, S., & Perry, A. (2009). Post-laryngectomy: It's hard to swallow: An Australian study of prevalence and self-reports of swallowing function after a total laryngectomy. *Dysphagia, 24*, 172–179.

Marcotte, P. (2006). *Critical review: Effectiveness of FEEs in comparison to VFSS at identifying aspiration*. Retrieved from https://www.uwo.ca/fhs/csd/ebp/reviews/2006-07/Marcotte.pdf.

McNeil, B. J., Weichselbaum, R., & Pauker, S. G. (1981). Speech and survival: Tradeoffs between quality and quantity of life in laryngeal cancer. *The New England Journal of Medicine, 305*(17), 982–987. doi:10.1056/NEJM198110223051704

Ogura, J. H., Marks, J. E., & Freeman, R. B. (1980). Results of conservation surgery for cancers of the supraglottis and pyriform sinus. *The Laryngoscope, 90,* 591–600.

O'Hara, J., Goff, D., Cocks, H., Moor, J., Hartley, C., Muirhead, C., & Patterson, J. (2016). One-year swallowing outcomes following transoral laser microsurgery +/- adjuvant therapy versus primary chemoradiotherapy for advanced stage oropharyngeal squamous cell carcinoma. *Clinical Otolaryngol, 41,* 169–175.

Ohmae, Y., Logemann, J. A., Kaiser, P., Hanson, D. G., & Kahrilas, P. J. (1996). Effects of two breath-holding maneuvers on oropharyngeal swallow. *The Annals of Otology, Rhinology, and Laryngology, 105*(2), 123–131.

Patterson, J., & Wilson, J. B. (2011). The clinical value of dysphagia preassessment in the management of head and neck cancer patients. *Current Opinion in Otolaryngology and Head and Neck Surgery, 19,* 177–181.

Rademaker, A. W., Logemann, J. A., Pauloski, B. R., Bowman, J. B., Lazarus, C. L., Sisson, G. A., ... Collins, S. L. (1993). Recovery of postoperative swallowing in patients undergoing partial laryngectomy. *Head Neck, 15,* 325–334.

Rosenthal, D. I., Mohamed, A. S., Weber, R. S., Garden, A. S., Sevak, P. R., Kies, M. S., . . . Fuller, C. D. (2015). Long-term outcomes after surgical or nonsurgical initial therapy for patients with T4 squamous cell carcinoma of the larynx: A 3-decade survey. *Cancer, 121*(10), 1608–1619. doi:10.1002/cncr.29241

Sasaki, C. T., Leder, S. B., Acton, L. M., & Maune, S. (2006). Comparison of the glottic closure reflex in traditional "open" versus endoscopic laser supraglottic laryngectomy. *Annals of Otolaryngology, Rhinology, and Laryngology, 115,* 93–96.

Scharpf, J., & Esclamado, J. M. (2003). Reconstruction with radial forearm flaps after ablative surgery for hypopharyngeal cancer. *Head Neck, 25,* 261–266.

Smith, J. C., Johnson, J. T., Cognetti, D. M., Landsittel, D. P., Gooding, W. E., Cano, E. R., & Myers, E. N. (2003). Quality of life, functional outcome, and costs of early glottic cancer. *The Laryngoscope, 113,* 68–76.

Stenson, K. M., Maccracken, E., Kunnavakkam, R., W Cohen, E. E., Portugal, L. D., Villaflor, V., ... Vokes, E. E. (2012). Chemoradiation for patients with large-volume laryngeal cancers. *Head & Neck, 34,* 1162–1167.

Stoeckli, S. J., Pawlik, A. B., & Lipp, M. (2000). Salvage surgery after failure of nonsurgical therapy for carcinoma of the larynx and hypopharynx. *Archives of Otolaryngology–Head & Neck Surgery, 126,* 1473–1477.

Suárez, C., Rodrigo, J. P., Silver, C. E., Hartl, D. M., Takes, R. P., Rinaldo, A., ... Ferlito, A. (2012). Laser surgery for early to moderately advanced glottic, supraglottic, and hypopharyngeal cancers. *Head Neck, 34,* 1028–1035.

Sweeny, L., Golden, J. B., White, H. N., Magnuson, J. S., Carroll, W. R., & Rosenthal, E. L. (2012). Incidence and outcomes of stricture formation postlaryngectomy. *Otolaryngology–Head and Neck Surgery, 146,* 395–402.

Timmermans, A. J., Lansaat, L., Theunissen, E. A., Hamming-Vrieze, O., Hilgers, F. J., & Van den brekel, M. W. (2014). Predictive factors for pharyngocutaneous fistulization after total laryngectomy. *Annals of Otolaryngology, Rhinology, and Laryngology, 123,* 153–161.

Wall, L. R., Ward, E. C., Cartmill, B., & Hill, A. J. (2013). Physiological changes to the swallowing mechanism following (chemo)radiotherapy for head and neck cancer: A systematic review. *Dysphagia, 28*(4), 481–493. doi:10.1007/s00455-013-9491-8

Ward, E. C., Bishop, B., Frisby, J., & Stevens, M. (2002). Swallowing outcomes following laryngectomy and pharyngolaryngectomy. *Archives of Otolaryngology–Head & Neck Surgery, 128,* 181–186.

Wasserman, T., Murry, T., Johnson, J. T., & Myers, E. N. (2001). Management of swallowing in supraglottic and extended supraglottic laryngectomy patients. *Head & Neck, 23*(12), 1043–1048. doi:10.1002/hed.1149

Welch, M. V., Logemann, J. A., Rademaker, A. W., & Kahrilas, P. J. (1993). Changes in pharyngeal dimensions effected by chin tuck. *Archives of Physical Medicine and Rehabilitation, 74*(2), 178–181.

Withrow, K. P., Rosenthal, E. L., Gourin, C. G., Peters, G. E., Magnus, J. S., Terris, D. J., & Carroll, W. W. (2007). Free tissue transfer to manage salvage laryngectomy defects after organ preservation failure. *The Laryngoscope, 117,* 781–784.

Wolf, G. T. (1991). Induction chemotherapy plus radiation compared with surgery plus radiation in patients with advanced laryngeal cancer. The Department of Veterans Affairs in Laryngeal Cancer Study Group. *New England Journal of Medicine, 324,* 1685–1690.

SUGGESTED READINGS

Alicandri-Ciufelli, M., Piccinini, A., Grammatica, A., Chiesi, A., Bergamini, G., Luppi, M. P., ... Presutti, L. (2013). Voice and swallowing after partial laryngectomy: Factors influencing outcome. *Head & Neck, 35,* 214–219.

Carrara-de Angelis, E., Feher, O., Barros, A. P. B., Nishimoto, I. N., & Kowalski, L. P. (2003). Voice and swallowing in patients enrolled in a larynx preservation trial. *Archives of Otolaryngology–Head & Neck Surgery, 129,* 733–738.

Francis, D. O., Weymuller, Ernest A., Jr., Parvathaneni, U., Merati, A. L., & Yueh, B. (2010). Dysphagia, stricture, and pneumonia in head and neck cancer patients: Does treatment modality matter? *Annals of Otology, Rhinology, and Laryngology, 119,* 391–397.

Haderlein, M., Semrau, S., Ott, O., Speer, S., Bohr, C., & Fietkau, R. (2014). Dose-dependent deterioration of swallowing function after induction chemotherapy and definitive chemoradiotherapy for laryngopharyngeal cancer. *Strahlentherapie Und Onkologie: Organ Der Deutschen Röntgengesellschaft ...[et al.], 190,* 192–198.

Jiang, N., Zhang, L., Li, L., Zhao, Y., & Eisele, D. W. (2014). Risk factors for late dysphagia after (chemo)radiotherapy for head and neck cancer: A systematic methodological review. *Head & Neck.* Advance online publication. doi:10.1002/hed.23963.

Maclean, J., Cotton, S., & Perry, A. (2008). Variation in surgical methods used for total laryngectomy in Australia. *Journal of Laryngology and Otolaryngology, 122,* 728–732.

Maruo, T., Fujimoto, Y., Ozawa, K., Hiramatsu, M., Suzuki, A., Nishio, N., & Nakashima, T. (2014). Laryngeal sensation and pharyngeal delay time after (chemo)radiotherapy. *European Archives of Oto-Rhino-Laryngology, 271,* 2299–2304.

Ozawa, K., Fujimoto, Y., & Nakashima, T. (2010). Changes in laryngeal sensation evaluated with a new method before and after radiotherapy. *European Archives of Oto-Rhino-Laryngology, 267,* 811–816.

Paleri, V., Roe, J. W. G., Strojan, P., Corry, J., Grégoire, V., Hamoir, M., ... Ferlito, A. (2014). Strategies to reduce long-term postchemoradiation dysphagia in patients with head and neck cancer: An evidence-based review. *Head & Neck, 36,* 431–443.

Patterson, J. M., McColl, E., Carding, P. N., Hildreth, A. J., Kelly, C., & Wilson, J. A. (2014). Swallowing in the first year after chemoradiotherapy for head and neck cancer: Clinician- and patient-reported outcomes. *Head & Neck, 36,* 352–358.

Pfister, D. G., Laurie, S. A., Weinstein, G. S., Mendenhall, W. M., Adelstein, D. J., Ang, K. K., ... Wolf, G. T. (2006). American society of clinical oncology clinical practice guideline for the use of larynx-preservation strategies in the treatment of laryngeal cancer. *Journal of Clinical Oncology, 24,* 3693–3704.

Portas, J., Socci, C. P., Scian, E. P., Queija Ddos, S., Ferreira, A. S., Dedivitis, R. A., & Barros, A. P. (2011). Swallowing after non-surgical treatment (radiation therapy/radiochemotherapy protocol) of laryngeal cancer. *Brazilian Journal of Otorhinolaryngology, 77,* 96–101.

Smith, J. C., Johnson, J. T., Cognetti, D. M., Landsittel, D. P., Gooding, W. E., Cano, E. R., & Myers, E. N. (2003). Quality of life, functional outcome, and costs of early glottic cancer. *The Laryngoscope, 113,* 68–76.

Strojan, P., Haigentz, M., Jr., Bradford, C. R., Wolf, G. T., Hartl, D. M., Langendijk, J. A., ... Ferlito, A. (2013). Chemoradiotherapy vs. total laryngectomy for primary treatment of advanced laryngeal squamous cell carcinoma. *Oral Oncology, 49,* 283–286.

Vokes, E. E. (2013). Competing roads to larynx preservation. *Journal of Clinical Oncology, 31,* 833–835.

7

Psychosocial Care of the Patient With Laryngeal Cancer

Katharine E. Duckworth, PhD and
Richard P. McQuellon, PhD

RATIONALE FOR PSYCHOSOCIAL CARE IN LARYNGEAL CANCER

The diagnosis and treatment of head and neck (HN) cancer is almost always an emotionally challenging experience because of the life-threatening nature of the disease and the possibility of physical changes and dysfunction (Devins, Otto, Irish, & Rodin, 2010; Moadel, Ostroff, & Schantz, 1998). Patients with HN cancer are at risk for many posttreatment psychological difficulties (Devins et al., 2010) and score high on distress measures relative to patients with other types of cancers (Singer et al., 2012; Zabora, BrintzenhofeSzoc, Curbow, Hooker, & Piantadosi, 2001). Within the HN classification of cancers, laryngeal cancer (LC) has associated psychosocial stressors and threats to quality of life (QOL), including partial or complete loss of voice, difficulty with swallowing, chewing, and communicating, and changes in body image and self-concept. The following is a list of interesting data from the National Cancer Institute (2015):

- There were an estimated 13,560 new cases and 3,640 deaths as a result of LC in 2015.

- There are approximately 90,000 survivors of LC currently living in the United States.

- Five-year relative survival rates range from a high of 75.9% for localized disease to a low of only 35.2% with distant disease.

- Although the median age at diagnosis is 66 years, 46.2% of patients with LC are between the ages of 45 and 64 years.

This chapter promotes an understanding of the complexities of providing counseling care for patients with LC and their families by doing the following:

Friberg, J. C., & Vinney, L. A.
Laryngeal Cancer: An Interdisciplinary
Resource for Practitioners (pp. 111-128).
© 2017 Taylor and Francis Group.

1. Providing an overview of the psychosocial consequences of LC, noting characteristics of those at increased risk for psychological morbidity, and describing a framework for psychosocial care

2. Describing a biopsychosocial model of understanding patients with HN cancer in general, and those with LC in particular, and listing interventions that can be used at a variety of time points along the survivorship trajectory from diagnosis through long-term survivorship

3. Focusing primarily on what we define as counseling interventions but recognizing that there are many other evidence-based psychosocial and integrative approaches (e.g., massage, acupuncture) that may alleviate the suffering of patients and their caregivers

4. Highlighting themes that patients might encounter along a three-phase survivorship trajectory and illustrating how they might be addressed in counseling with a case study

There are a host of concerns (e.g., loss of social/professional roles, fear of recurrence, grief) that are more or less problematic for patients with LC depending on the psychological resources and social supports available for each individual patient. These resources can be internal or external and might include the following:

- Optimism

- Resilience

- Realistic expectations about cancer treatment(s) and outcome(s)

- Overall health literacy

- Financial resources/support

- Knowledgeable caregivers

- Faith/church communities

- Social media (e.g., caringbridge.com)

Our review of the research on psychosocial problems and QOL deficits was selective. We have attempted to cite relevant research where it will highlight a clinical issue of importance. We describe how our psychosocial oncology group is situated within the broader health care team to provide mental health care services in a dynamic setting. Finally, we reference behavior change methods and resources to address maladaptive behaviors such as smoking. Our hope is to inform health care providers from a variety of disciplines about the psychosocial needs of patients and family members and offer methods for reducing suffering and improving patient QOL.

BIOPSYCHOSOCIAL MODEL OF CARE

A biopsychosocial model of multidisciplinary care for patients with cancer combines medically focused patient-centered care (Epstein & Street, 2007) with the integration of mental health and other allied health care professionals at all levels (Engel, 1977). Thus, with this model of care, the body and mind are targeted in combination with the patient and important other members of the LC care team. This model is useful when considering patients with HN cancer, because they can present with a host of biological, psychological, and social problems that result from their disease and/or treatment(s). A biopsychosocial model of care enables a deeper understanding of a patient's situation from all practitioners that leads to action. The model also holds that health or illness outcomes are a consequence of the relationship between biological, psychological, and social factors that operate within (microlevel) and outside (macrolevel) a patient at any given time (Wilson & Cleary, 1995). For example, attending to the psychological and social aspects of a patient's life can direct attention to macrolevel processes such as the presence of a helpful caregiver or a supportive employer. The presence or absence of caregiver support can interact with microlevel events such as poor nutrition. An inability to gain adequate nourishment via oral or tube feedings can result in malnutrition in a patient with LC. This patient may subsequently experience fatigue, mild depression, and/or waning social support as a result of the loss of normal function before and after treatment. The presence of a supportive caregiver can alleviate these issues; however, the absence of such support can have the opposite effect.

The biopsychosocial model takes health and illness into account and provides the conceptual framework for understanding patient adaptation after rigorous medical treatments. In the previous example, the biopsychosocial approach directs providers to inquire about caloric intake and social support in the home, perhaps leading to both a medical intervention (e.g., medications to increase appetite and/or nutritional supplements) and a behavioral intervention (e.g., caregiver/physician/speech-language pathologist [SLP] consultation to improve nutritional sufficiency).

HEALTH-RELATED QUALITY OF LIFE

The diagnosis and treatment of HN cancer may interrupt and impair the QOL of patients, at least for a time. Health-related quality of life (HR-QOL) refers to the extent to which one's usual or expected physical, emotional, social/family, and functional well-being are affected by a medical condition or its treatment (Cella & Bonomi, 1995). There are psychometrically sound paper-and-pencil self-report instruments that can measure HR-QOL accurately and inform providers about fluctuations in HR-QOL throughout treatment (Trask, Hsu, & McQuellon, 2009). Factors that affect patient-reported QOL and adaptation to HN cancer are numerous and may include the following (Devins et al., 2010):

- Premorbid characteristics of the patient (e.g., socioeconomic status, functional status, dispositional optimism)

- Tumor site

- Adverse treatment effects (e.g., issues with speech, feeding problems, chronic dry mouth, taste disturbance)

- Smoking

- Problem drinking

- Pain

- Depression

- Fear of recurrence

Factors that affect QOL also can be thought of as risk factors for poor psychosocial outcomes. In other words, a patient who presents with a number of factors that can affect his or her QOL might have a harder time returning to pretreatment levels of psychosocial function than others. Consider a patient who demonstrates complex communication needs and who also scores low on dispositional optimism, has few social supports, and is of low socioeconomic status. This patient may be at greater risk for anxiety and depression than a patient with fewer risk factors. That said, the findings from one study suggested that QOL returns to pretreatment levels approximately 1 year after treatment for surviving patients (Griffiths, Parmar, & Bailey, 1999), although it depends entirely on individual and unique patient needs, functional status, and environmental situations.

Because risk factors alone cannot define a patient's need for counseling and emotional support, evidence and a solid rationale exist for using patient-rated outcome measures (PROs), such as screening, to improve cancer care (Kotronoulas et al., 2014). A PRO can facilitate improved communication between physicians and patients and lead to higher patient satisfaction and an improved sense of control. One group of researchers retrospectively examined PRO symptom questionnaires exclusively from patients with LC (Rinkel et al., 2014). They focused on voice, speech, and swallowing, all of which are crucial functional capacities that directly affect valued activities such as sharing a meal with friends. The researchers concluded that, after treatment, the prevalence of voice, speech, and swallowing problems is high and related to overall QOL and reported distress levels. They also observed a disconnect in what the patients reported, because only 8% of the respondents expressed a need for speech and swallowing rehabilitation after treatment despite clinically significant scores on instrumental measures of voice, speech, and swallowing deficits that indicated a need for remediation. The authors speculated that these findings were linked to limited health literacy and the likelihood that such patients got "lost" in the health care system. Another explanation might be that, because patients were assessed from 3 months to 5 years after treatment, they had made peace with their respective losses or functional changes rather than seeking ways to address them.

Treatment of Laryngeal Cancer and Quality of Life

Most patients in the early decision-making process may assume that sparing the larynx would be optimal under any circumstances and result in a better QOL. However, choosing chemoradiation therapy (CRT) over surgery does not guarantee better QOL in the long run. Specifically, patients who have undergone CRT for HN cancer have indicated variable QOL, across time, as a function of comorbidity, tumor site, and survival. Thus, a host of risk factors and protective resources (e.g., diagnosis-related, personal, biological, psychological, physical, lifestyle-related, and social factors) exist that combine to predict QOL (Devins et al., 2010). In addition, clinical experience suggests that patients who have chronic difficulty swallowing might regret laryngeal preservation via CRT or other treatments, because once a patient is impaired, swallowing may be valued more than voice.

Patients who pursue surgical treatment for LC experience QOL concerns, as well, which can affect their overall psychosocial functioning. For example, after partial or total laryngectomy, patients may feel that their sense of identity has been altered radically because of loss of voice and other communication/feeding impairments. In addition, because surgical options are often sought for more advanced LCs, a partial or total laryngectomy may be associated with fear for the future (e.g., recurrence of cancer, death), which can contribute to a patient's psychological distress. Postlaryngectomy speech therapy may help alleviate some of this distress in relationship to communication experiences (Pereira da Silva, Feliciano, Vaz Freitas, Esteves, & Almeida E Sousa, 2015). Thus, both psychological evaluation/treatment and speech therapy are recommended after laryngectomy to address specific patient needs and concerns (Pereira da Silva et al., 2015).

CENTRALITY OF VOICE AND APPEARANCE

Voice and physical appearance are central to psychological and emotional well-being. For patients after treatments for LC, the phrase "I am not myself" might hold true until they can adjust to physical and concomitant psychological changes that accompany both medical and surgical treatment approaches. Cooley (1902) created the concept of the looking-glass self, which suggests that a person's self emerges out of interpersonal interactions and the perceptions of others. According to Cooley, we see ourselves literally become ourselves, through the eyes of others. Using the looking-glass self as a model for self-identity, the following questions emerge when a patient encounters a negative reaction from others after radical HN surgery:

- What happens to a person who is greeted regularly with quizzical or critical appraisals by others?

Box 7-1

Former poet laureate Ted Kooser and contemporary singer John Prine both had LC and subsequent treatment that affected their voices. In their situations, loss of voice may have meant the loss of their profession. Fortunately, both of them made an excellent recovery and ended up reflecting on their story on stage at the Library of Congress (http://www.loc.gov/today/cyberlc/feature_wdesc.php?rec=3677).

- What happens to a person who is the focal point of stares from others as an initial reaction to his or her postsurgical appearance (Garland-Thomson, 2009)?

- How would such interactions influence a person's sense of self?

- Is the emotional reaction to loss of voice even more pronounced for those who have experienced previous societal marginalization on account of race, sex, sexual orientation, or any other number of characteristics?

A person's voice may also be integral to his or her sense of identity. Reaction to its permanent loss may range from catastrophic to problematic depending on a host of circumstances. Compromise of QOL as a result of voice loss will depend on whether a person uses his or her voice for consistent vocational and social communication or is relatively quiet (Box 7-1).

Radical voice and appearance changes can create stigma and engender patient self-blame and/or shame. Physical stigma that results from disfigurement can be felt deeply and become disruptive to a person's social world. Because nicotine and alcohol use are risk factors for HN cancers, patients who are diagnosed with LC may be at risk for bouts of destructive self-blame and regret over the past. Because of self-blame, shame, and other resulting emotions, it is imperative that the multidisciplinary treatment team look at each patient in a kind, nonjudgmental manner and listen carefully to his or her story. Doing so will help patients find their voice again so that they may rediscover or preserve their place in the social fabric of life.

PSYCHOSOCIAL ASSESSMENT, REFERRAL, AND COUNSELING WITH PATIENTS WITH LARYNGEAL CANCER

Thorough psychosocial assessment is necessary in the early stages of cancer treatment because it can help the treatment team identify the need for counseling and anticipate problems over the course of care. Patients' emotional responses to the stress of initial diagnosis and treatment vary widely. Thus, acquiring an individualized view of each patient's psychosocial status is critical (Derogatis et al., 1983). For those who struggle with psychosocial aspects of their diagnosis, counseling is likely to be beneficial.

Counseling is generally thought of as a verbal interaction between a trained professional and a patient. In cancer care, this interaction often includes the patient's caregivers or family members. Depending on the stage and nature of the surgical or medical interventions, patients with LC may be unable to produce voice, or their vocal quality may be compromised and affect speech intelligibility. Thus, professionals may need to adapt traditional counseling to enable the patient to participate fully. That said, counseling is only one method of psychosocial care among a variety of possibilities. Other options include pharmacotherapy, music therapy, massage, healing touch, expressive therapies, pastoral care, and community educational and support options, all of which may be more or less useful on the basis of the characteristics of the patient and his or her place along the diagnostic and treatment trajectory.

In reference to counseling, a *psychosocial oncology counselor* (a psychology professional with expertise in psychosocial oncology) who is familiar with HN cancer and its attendant challenges is the best source of help for patients and their family and/or caregivers. Informal counseling is often delivered by a host of professional caregivers (occupational therapists, physical therapists, SLPs, nurses, physicians, etc.) and nonprofessional caregivers (family members, friends, and veteran patients) involved in the multidisciplinary care of patients. Providing basic training in counseling skills or doctor-patient communication skill training can help professional helpers who are not specialists in psychosocial oncology make a difference in the lives of patients and their family members (Back, Arnold, Tulsky, Baile, & Fryer-Edwards, 2003). That said, we recommend that best practice/standard of care include a consultation from a psychosocial oncology counselor coupled with more informal multidisciplinary team involvement for all patients with LC. The most common type of intervention delivered by an oncology counselor is supportive counseling, which consists of the following (Wills, 1991):

- Deep listening
- Emotional support
- Information giving
- Help with tasks (e.g., managing insurance difficulties)
- Social companionship

Although some of these functions overlap and can be provided by loving, thoughtful family members, deep listening is a characteristic of professional counseling that is not commonly found in most informal caregiver networks. Specifically, psychosocial oncology counselors are trained specifically to listen thoughtfully and respond during a spontaneous human interaction while at the same time maintaining some emotional distance from the patient. Good candidates for standard talk therapy beyond the initial consultation are people who have some measure of distress, are curious about how they might change their situation, and report that they benefit from talking about what is on their mind. People who have been members of a support group, such as Alcoholics Anonymous, often are accustomed to the level of self-disclosure that is common in counseling. Therefore, they are likely to benefit from a referral for counseling.

A psychosocial oncology counselor needs to be mindful of the timing of any intervention and be informed about effective evidence-based means of working with patients along the trajectory of their LC experience. Both research and clinical experience have demonstrated that patients find different things important during early- vs late-stage care (Metcalfe, Lowe, & Rogers, 2014). For example, patients who are in the middle of a course of intensive radiotherapy treatment may be preoccupied with impaired speech or other symptoms (e.g., anxiety, pain, fatigue), whereas as they adapt to their new normal, they may be more concerned about swallowing problems and the reality of permanent loss of function. Awareness of these concerns and the three-phase trajectory of survivorship for patients with LC (Table 7-1) can be helpful in treatment planning.

Screenings for Psychosocial Distress

Health care providers tend to under-report the psychological distress of patients with cancer as a result of too little training in biopsychosocial assessment and the patients' reluctance to discuss their feelings (Fisch et al., 2003; Laugsand et al., 2010; Passik et al., 1998). As a result, the Institute of Medicine's Committee on Cancer and the American College of Surgeons promoted guidelines that require regular distress screening for all cancer survivors as part of a patient-centered survivorship care plan (Institute of Medicine, 2008). This policy should result in more psychological care for patients with HN cancer after treatment at a time when QOL deficits and permanent losses of structure and/or function might become burdensome.

TABLE 7-1
THEMES, TASKS, AND PSYCHOSOCIAL ISSUES IN THE THREE STAGES OF LARYNGEAL CANCER TREATMENT

STAGE OF TREATMENT	COMMON THEMES, TASKS, AND PSYCHOSOCIAL ISSUES ACCORDING TO STAGE
1. Pretreatment decision making and preparation	• Considering alternative treatments • Managing the uncertainty of treatment outcome • Confronting mortality and self-blame* (e.g., "I did this to myself by smoking") • Financial considerations/insurance limitations • Informed-consent process • Symptoms of anxiety, depression, and distress*
2. Active treatment intervention	• Adopting the patient role in the inpatient (surgical) or outpatient (radiation/chemotherapy) setting • Managing acute treatment side effects • Confronting unfamiliar procedures and treatment (e.g., nasogastric or percutaneous endoscopic gastrostomy tube placement) • Adjusting to altered body image • Heightened physical and emotional vulnerability • Maintaining morale and hope; managing discouragement • Dealing with complications
3. Adaptation to functional changes and the "new normal"	• Accepting permanent losses (e.g., loss of natural voice) and the possibility of long-term effects • Contending with the stress of ongoing medical appointments • Learning to "live with, lessen, or lose" a symptom or adverse effect of treatment • Recovery of valued roles in community and at work and home • Encountering regret over treatment decision making (e.g., "buyer's remorse") • Complying with self-care, including recommendations to discontinue drinking and smoking • Reestablishing primary identity/relinquishing patient role

*Many of these issues continue over the course of care. For example, confronting mortality and the episodes of fear of recurrence may be revisited more or less intensely each time the patient returns for follow-up care. Anxiety, depressive symptoms, and distress may emerge over the three stages.

In addition to regular screenings to ascertain the psychosocial status of patients, suicide assessments might be relevant for this population, because the rate of suicide tends to be higher in patients with HN cancer than in those with other diagnoses (Misono, Weiss, Fann, Redman, & Yueh, 2008). Patients who express active suicidal ideation and/or intent to harm themselves must be assessed promptly and referred to a psychosocial oncology counselor and/or psychiatrist in a timely manner.

STAGES OF TREATMENT FOR LARYNGEAL CANCER

The previous sections discuss the benefits of counseling for patients with LC and explain reasons that patients might be in need of psychosocial support from their health care providers. The next section explains differentiated patient needs with regard to counseling across three distinct stages of treatment for LC:

- Stage 1: pretreatment decision making and preparation
- Stage 2: active treatment intervention
- Stage 3: adaptation to functional changes and the "new normal"

Each of these stages is outlined in Table 7-1 and described in depth here.

Stage 1: Pretreatment Decision Making and Preparation

Patients in the first stage of LC treatment, pretreatment decision making and preparation, are tasked with coming to some understanding of their condition and how it will affect their immediate future. At this time, health care providers can assess their patients' unique combination of coping skills, past treatment experiences, and social supports to determine whether they are more or less vulnerable to a wide range of adjustment problems, which can include the following:

- Anxiety
- Depression
- Sleep disturbance
- Body image concerns
- Interruption of valued life roles
- Intimacy concerns
- Low health literacy
- Inaccurate treatment expectations

As noted earlier, a thorough assessment of patients' psychological status and support resources is crucial. Patients with HN cancer often confront specific problems on account of the location of and prognosis for their disease as well as the multimodal treatments they may undergo.

At the time of initial diagnosis, allied health care providers will likely encounter patients contending with a wider range of physical symptoms and the anticipation of specific problems depending on the information they receive. A dismal prognosis can trigger a host of psychosocial stressors including intense distress, fear of death, and anticipatory loss (Moadel et al., 1998). Although HN cancers can be diagnosed in anyone, there is an increased incidence in male smokers over the age of 50 years with a history of alcohol consumption (Devins et al., 2010; Moadel et al., 1998). Patients with this profile may be hesitant to use counseling or participate in substance-cessation offerings. They might also suffer from other comorbid disorders that can affect their psychosocial wellness (Devins et al., 2010). Patients are often confronted with the need to make

---

Box 7-2

Our psychosocial oncology group at Wake Forest Baptist Medical Center provides both inpatient and outpatient consultation in an academic medical center (McQuellon, Hurt, & DeChatelet, 1996). Patients may be initially self-referred or identified from any number of the staff or health care team, including physical therapists, surgeons, SLPs, nurses, medical oncologists, and other allied health professionals. Our team is administratively located within the hematology/oncology section and has a suite of offices located adjacent to medical, surgical, and radiation oncology services. This setup allows us to respond quickly to the results of consultations received from the surgical or radiation oncology teams and to see patients in a variety of settings, which results in psychosocial care that is integrated throughout treatment. Patients may be seen in their hospital room, outpatient treatment pod, or clinical follow-up appointment. We also use other resources available within our medical center (e.g., chaplains, massage therapists, therapeutic music) and in the broader community (e.g., acupuncture, tai chi).

---

critical decisions about their care quickly after being given a dizzying array of information about treatment and adverse effects. Although the number of treatment and reconstructive options have increased over the years, the possibility of confronting treatment outcomes that yield long-term QOL impairment remains an all-too-real possibility. The prevalence of depression is high at diagnosis, in active treatment, and for the 6 months after treatment (Chen et al., 2013; Haisfield-Wolfe, McGuire, Soeken, Geiger-Brown, & De Forge, 2009). Certain variables, such as marital status, education, symptom burden, and positioning within the illness trajectory affect these depression rates. In addition, current depression burden often predicts future depression burden (Haisfield-Wolfe et al., 2009). High rates of distress (Zabora et al., 2001) and suicide completion have been reported in patients with cancer. Specifically, the suicide rate for people with LC is 46.8/100,000 persons (Misono et al., 2008). For this reason, patient and caregiver education is an important part of stage 1 LC treatment.

The provision of information and appropriate teaching about upcoming changes in appearance, functional status, and self-care is critical, especially when treatments can result in significant physical changes (Moadel et al., 1998). Health care providers should provide information to patients recently diagnosed with LC regarding the following:

- Coping with the effects of multimodal treatment
- The impact of treatment on basic functions of living (e.g., breathing, swallowing, and communicating)
- Supportive interventions aimed to assist with coping

We strongly recommend standard-of-care "prehabilitation" or pretreatment education to help patients develop informed expectations regarding their treatments. Many patients cannot fully understand what lies ahead until they actually experience it, and as a result, they may have unrealistic expectations about posttreatment outcomes (Andrykowski et al., 1995). When these expectations are not fulfilled, additional psychological distress may be experienced (Box 7-2).

To exemplify the concerns most often noted in stage 1 of LC treatment, consider Mr. Grant, a hypothetical patient featured in the following section as a three-part case study. Case Study 7-1 demonstrates how an oncology counselor might initially work with a patient diagnosed with LC. This case illustrates many of the tasks and psychosocial challenges that patients with HN cancer face.

CASE STUDY 7-1

PATIENT NAME: MR. GRANT

Clinical Status: immediately after diagnosis of LC

Mr. Grant is a 58-year-old man diagnosed with stage T3, N0, M0 right-sided laryngeal squamous cell carcinoma. He had numerous biopsies on his right vocal cord before a final diagnosis was made, which was a source of irritation and anxiety for him and his spouse, who wondered why the medical team could not hurry up and make treatment recommendations. Mr. Grant and his wife were heavy users of the Internet and frightened by what they learned about treatment morbidity and survival statistics. Mr. Grant was stunned by the information on treatment duration and short- and long-term toxicities, the possibility of him needing a percutaneous endoscopic gastrostomy (PEG) tube, his potential need for a tracheostomy, the likelihood that he would need to stop work for a time, his possible need for dental care, and the directive to stop smoking immediately or risk poor treatment outcomes. This information was overwhelming and triggered panic-like attacks in him. Mr. Grant was referred for management of his anxiety and was seen for two sessions of supportive counseling (on information giving and emotional support) and guided imagery/relaxation training to help reduce anxiety just before the initiation of his CRT. He reported reduced anxiety and less fear about the future as he began therapy. He said that he would call for additional help as needed.

Stage 2: Active Treatment Intervention

After patients have made critical treatment decisions, they may experience escalating distress in the anticipatory pretreatment phase as the day of their treatment approaches. The active treatment and recovery phases can bring additional challenges, including coping with long hospital stays or medical complications, second thoughts about treatment choices/decisions, physical withdrawal from nicotine or alcohol, pain management, familial distress, and disruption of thyroid function resulting in hormonally induced depression (Moadel et al., 1998). For example, the patient who learns that his chance of survival with laryngectomy is only slightly better than that with radiotherapy may struggle in making a treatment decision. Likewise, the patient who elects radiotherapy to preserve vocal function may encounter difficulty swallowing or find that the voice is impaired as a result of treatment effects. In contrast, the sudden loss of voice after laryngectomy may be devastating. Although the daily grind of radiotherapy can be exhausting, the sudden impact of surgery can be shocking. We turn again to Mr. Grant as an exemplar of how counseling can support a patient in stage 2 of LC treatment (Case Study 7-2).

Stage 3: Adaptation to Functional Changes and the "New Normal"

As patients transition out of the active medical treatment phase and move toward stage 3 of LC treatment, the entire health care team, and psychosocial oncology counselors in particular, should support patients as they monitor for signs of recurrence and any fear of recurrence that impairs their social, professional, and/or personal functioning. Other concerns that patients identify at this stage are financial distress, role reintegration, residual communication challenges, depression, compromised self-esteem, and intimacy issues (Moadel et al., 1998).

Voice loss affects patients uniquely on the basis of their personal disposition, their coping mechanisms, and the role that voice plays in their daily routines. Alternative forms of communication,

---

CASE STUDY 7-2

PATIENT NAME: MR. GRANT

Clinical Status: 4 months after treatment

Mr. Grant had a very difficult treatment course. Radiation therapy led to immobility and atrophy of his vocal folds, which resulted in compromised vocal function. During the middle of his course of radiation therapy, he reported feeling helpless because of the treatment effects coupled with the need to interrupt his normal work/travel schedule. He also was distressed by mucositis and dysphagia, which hampered his social life. In particular, he stopped dining out with friends as he had typically done in the past. Mr. Grant's dysphagia eventually necessitated the placement of a PEG tube. Although the PEG tube was all but unnoticeable by most observers, he felt acutely uncomfortable with it. He had a history of smoking and alcohol and cocaine abuse that led him to make self-critical statements (e.g., "I did this to myself"). Counseling consisted of six sessions. The focus of these sessions was strategizing how to best adapt to his changing role at work, lack of energy, and self-consciousness about the sound of his voice and the appearance of his PEG tube.

Mr. Grant had always been exceptionally social and, although he was deeply depressed by his medical situation, was still able to make engaging comments to many of his health care providers. His radiation oncology technicians, radiation therapist, and consulting surgeon enjoyed working with him and spoke with him at length. He responded well to this ongoing form of incidental counseling and encouragement.

Daily radiation treatments and chemotherapy left Mr. Grant fatigued. He became increasingly socially isolated and lonely. He refused to attend his church because of his appearance and inability to communicate well, which was a source of frustration to his wife, who tried to encourage him. Because he was unable to eat for a time, he chose to not engage in his customary social activities, such as lunch with some of his sales partners. They were quite supportive of him initially, but over time, their contacts diminished. With work gone, only church remained.

---

including lip reading, alternative and augmentative communication, alaryngeal speech modes, and the use of writing and creative expression, may be used in the clinical encounter to facilitate meaningful communication. Supportive community groups can be a powerful source of healing and support and also can supplement a patient or caregiver's knowledge base and social system (Box 7-3).

Finally, caregivers and significant others likely will need support as they adjust to new routines after treatment; high distress levels, restlessness, and a need for additional relaxation strategies in spouses of laryngectomees have been reported (Meyer et al., 2015). For patients with a poor prognosis, end-of-life care considerations become pertinent in Stage 3, as well. Such considerations include practical (e.g., advance directives/living wills, financial arrangements) and existential support that is needed when confronting death, as can be seen in the continuation of Mr. Grant's case in Case Study 7-3.

It should be noted that Mr. Grant is a fictional composite of many patients, and his case study is intended to emphasize issues that can emerge in each stage from diagnosis through the end of treatment. Patients and family members are often so busy with medical appointments and disruptive physical side-effects that they have little time for yet one more appointment; thus, they might be candidates for counseling months after treatment ends when the reality of their losses and deficits sets in and the constant support of nurses, physicians, physician assistants, and SLPs is waning. Posttreatment let-down is common in cancer care (Hurt, McQuellon, & Barrett, 1994).

Box 7-3

A support group used locally by our psychosocial oncology team is a laryngectomy group called "The Western Piedmont Speak Easy" support group. It is designed for laryngectomees, their families, and caregivers and offers a friendly and supportive atmosphere and provides information about living without a voice, including where to find supplies and how to manage unique medical issues (e.g., stoma and postsurgical care).

Case Study 7-3

PATIENT NAME: MR. GRANT

Clinical Status: 1 year after treatment

The posttreatment adjustment period after active medical treatment was very difficult for Mr. Grant. While his medical treatment was successful, it left him with significant impairments and quality-of-life deficits. He became intensely depressed and developed feelings of helplessness and hopelessness. These feelings were intensified because his compromised voice and need for tube feedings persisted long after treatment had ended. He was seen a total of 10 times for counseling. His inability to speak well eventually resulted in the loss of his job as a pharmaceutical salesman, which was extremely disheartening to him. In addition, he had several severe psychosocial stressors, including the loss of his home to foreclosure.

His counseling was challenging, because Mr. Grant was very frustrated by his inability to speak easily and fluently. He could barely whisper. Thus, the counseling itself, which requires a verbal exchange, was a reminder of his loss and disability. However, the assumed temporary nature of his voice impairment was a source of hope for him. "I can do almost anything if I know it will be over someday," he would say. He was aphonic for a time and often needed to write his responses in the counseling sessions. Nevertheless, he proceeded successfully through biweekly counseling meetings and adjusted to his significant voice impairment and overall quality-of-life decline (e.g., he could no longer enjoy a cigar or an alcoholic drink).

Mr. Grant's counselor was trained in the specialty of psychosocial oncology and made use of supportive and problem-solving counseling and self-talk. When Mr. Grant would become down on his situation or have negative, intrusive thoughts ("what's the use, it's going to come back anyway"), his counselor would ask him to use his own words in response (i.e., "I can get through anything ... this will pass") and to develop a set of positive responses. This took some training and work, because Mr. Grant had a "glass is half-empty" approach to life. He was given a list of supportive care and survivorship activities (massage, acupuncture, support groups) that were available at the cancer center at which he was treated and in the community where he lived.

The prominent themes in his counseling sessions were loss (voice, job, social activities, health), angry guilt ("Look what I did to myself!"), and fear of recurrence. His self-blame regarding smoking was not a motivator for him to quit. He was able only to cut down by about 50% to half of a pack/day, although he no longer drank alcohol or used illicit drugs. He had an excellent relationship with his surgeon and his SLP, who facilitated feelings of hopefulness in him.

(continued)

CASE STUDY 7-3 (CONTINUED)

Mr. Grant was evaluated at a voice and swallowing disorders clinic 1 year after completion of his treatment. His chronic mucosal irritation was treated with over-the-counter "magic" mouth wash. He noted continued difficulty swallowing and the feeling that food was stuck in his throat. He was subsequently referred for surgical intervention to improve his overall voice and swallowing function. He also saw an SLP, who helped him improve his swallow function. The ongoing chronic nature of his problems was a nagging source of stress for Mr. Grant, and he subsequently experienced recurrent periods of depressive affect. However, with periodic counseling sessions with a psychosocial oncology specialist, he was able to make an adequate adjustment to his chronic QOL deficits.

Although our case study does not highlight end-of-life issues, it should be noted that people with advanced disease might actually encounter such concerns at diagnosis. These patients are good candidates for intensive work with psychosocial oncology and palliative care professionals. These members of the health care team can provide pain management, support increased QOL, and facilitate team-based care for patients with LC (see Chapter 8 for more information on palliative care specialists).

EVIDENCE BASE FOR PSYCHOSOCIAL INTERVENTIONS

There is a small but significant amount of literature on clinical interventions designed to address psychological problems of an improved QOL for patients with HN cancer. Psychosocial interventions in this population can be both feasible and efficacious, especially those that are part of routine care. The Nurse Counseling and After Intervention program is one of a few randomized controlled psychosocial interventions that have reported both short- and long-term results for patients (van der Meulen et al., 2014). Specifically, the following aspects of counseling care were found to produce positive outcomes:

- Regularly scheduled counseling sessions
- Evaluation and discussion of interpersonal relationships
- Conversations focused on fear of recurrence, hypermonitoring, and personal cancer perceptions/beliefs

In one study, those who received counseling services focused on these bullet points experienced improved physical and emotional functioning, diminished pain, fewer problems with swallowing and mouth opening, and diminished depressive symptoms. In addition, formal counseling led to long-term effects such as the following (Humphris & Ozakinci, 2008; van der Meulen et al., 2014):

- Improved global QOL
- Increased ability to perform important life roles
- Improved emotional functioning
- Decreased pain
- Decreased swallowing and chewing difficulties
- Reductions in depressive symptoms

Such findings reveal the potential for clinical interventions to have significant positive effects on HR-QOL and depressive symptoms within this population.

Formal counseling is not always easily accessible for patients with LC. In some cases, this lack of access can compromise or affect the frequency and length of counseling interventions. Many patients in rural locations must travel long distances for treatment and follow-up care. For this reason, telephone-based interventions may be an economical and practical method of care. For example, in one study, eight sessions of a telephone-based coping and stress-management intervention timed strategically to coincide with key points along the care continuum resulted in reductions in distress for patients with LC (Kilbourn et al., 2013). In addition, these patients reported satisfaction with and self-efficacy in their ability to apply the skills learned during the intervention. Despite these results, the feasibility and desirability of telephone-based interventions for patients with limited voice remain undetermined.

Luckett, Britton, Clover, and Rankin (2011) performed a systematic review of the evidence in support of psychological interventions with patients with HN cancer and concluded that the most support exists for psychoeducational efforts that provide counseling and patient education simultaneously (Luckett et al., 2011). Although the studies to date have been compelling in their support for counseling as an impactful part of LC care, additional attention is needed to extend the current research base in this area via studies that have the following characteristics (Kilbourn et al., 2013; Luckett et al., 2011; van der Meulen et al., 2014):

- Be randomized and controlled
- Document effect sizes
- Adhere to treatment measures for research efficacy
- Explore interventions that coincide with routine care
- Include patient participants with high distress
- Be multicentered trials with significant sample sizes
- Include diverse people
- Focus on the development of theoretically based interventions

HEALTHY BEHAVIORS AND LARYNGEAL CANCER

As a component of psychosocial counseling occurring as part of routine LC care, many counselors advise patients about healthy behaviors to support treatment and recovery. It is fortunate that most people with a diagnosis of LC are candidates for interventions designed to facilitate the reduction of tobacco usage, modify dietary preferences on the basis of personal taste and physiological function, and develop regular exercise habits. Through the modification and adoption of existing and new health habits, both survival and QOL may be maximized (Ligibel, 2012).

Smoking Behavior

Those who previously smoked tobacco may continue to face a higher relative risk of LC recurrence than do nonsmokers. However, a review of epidemiological studies found that the risk of LC is reduced within years after cessation and continues to decrease over time (Bosetti, Garavello, Gallus, & La, 2006). Specifically, a 60% reduction in risk has been noted 10 to 15 years after cessation, and a further decline is observed 20 years afterward. Thus, it benefits all health care providers to be aware of methods for smoking cessation. Some researchers have highlighted the interrelated nature of smoking, alcohol usage, and depression and, therefore, the efficacy of common treatments for these presenting concerns. Duffy et al. (2006) found that patients with HN cancer who were provided intervention consisting of cognitive-behavioral therapy and medication were significantly more likely to stop smoking and experience decreased symptoms of depression.

The authors suggested that treating these comorbidities together, rather than individually, may be more practical and might result in increased smoking-cessation rates.

Nutrition

Nutritional support and exercise interventions also have been examined within this population, predominantly with a focus on encouraging increases in nutritional intake. One study found that the use of an appetite stimulant might help patients maintain weight over the course of curative radiotherapy of the head and neck or lung and can improve specific aspects of QOL (McQuellon et al., 2002). A systematic review of patients with HN cancer who received radiotherapy revealed the possible utility of dietary counseling, prophylactic *enteral nutrition*, and appetite stimulants; however, the authors called for more prospective randomized trials related to nutrition within this population and noted the limitations of their findings that resulted from a lack of comparison groups and examinations of these approaches in combination (Garg, Yoo, & Winquist, 2010). The ideal means of providing nutritional support to patients with HN cancer who are undergoing various treatments warrants additional research.

Exercise

Health care providers also play a role in encouraging patients to incorporate exercise in their daily routine. It is possible that the stage or extent of disease, rather than the diagnosis itself, may be more impactful on exercise patterns because of the radical treatments that might be needed for those with more extensive disease. In a systematic review of randomized and controlled clinical trials of patients with cancer before and after medical intervention, physical exercise was found to have a positive effect on physiology, HR-QOL, performance measures, patient-reported functioning and symptoms, and emotional well-being (Knols, Aaronson, Uebelhart, Fransen, & Aufdemkampe, 2005). These beneficial effects may be moderated by the lifestyle choices of the patient, stage of the disease, and treatment modalities chosen; however, the potential positive implications of physical activity are sufficient to warrant encouragement from all health care providers. The results of one review of the exercise patterns of patients with HN cancer indicated that few of them engaged in moderate-to-vigorous exercise, and more than 50% of the respondents were entirely sedentary. In those patients who did exercise, the total number of minutes spent exercising has been associated with improvement in QOL ratings and fatigue (Rogers et al., 2006).

Many patients with HN cancer may be in need of education, encouragement, and even suggestions about specific exercise opportunities. McNeely et al. (2008) examined the role of progressive resistance exercise training (PRET) within this population. They reported significantly reduced shoulder pain and disability and enhanced endurance and upper-extremity muscular strength in patients with HN cancer who participated in PRET after surgery (McNeely et al., 2008). Such resistance training can be a beneficial component of postsurgical rehabilitation for certain patients with HN cancer.

CONCLUSION

The central issue for patients who are dealing with HN cancer, and LC in particular, is temporary or permanent loss of function. The manifestations of adjustment to loss of voice, albeit temporary or permanent, can be varied. Most if not all patients with HN cancer can benefit from brief, empowering, and motivating interactions from health care providers across all stages of their cancer, from diagnosis through treatment. This incidental counseling is delivered by various health care providers in the form of encouragement, information giving, empathy, and coaching. This chapter can serve as a resource for helpers from various backgrounds and as a template for understanding many of the common themes and challenges that patients face throughout treatment.

The largest challenge faced by many practitioners is recognizing the patients in need of psychosocial counseling and connecting them to the appropriate resources that can be integrated into their broader medical care. It is an art to successfully refer patients who need and want a form of traditional counseling to manage anxiety and depression to qualified providers (Worden & Weisman, 1980). The effective psychosocial oncology counselor will remain mindful of the dynamic medical landscape and treatment choices patients with HN cancer confront, guide patients and caregivers on their journeys, and work collaboratively with providers from other disciplines to enhance QOL throughout the continuum of treatment. They may also promote healthy behaviors and refer select patients to available interventions that address voice loss and other functional status impairments (e.g., swallowing, eating, respiration). The effects of LC are far-reaching and require time and effort to manage. With that in mind, regaining functions such as communicating, swallowing, and breathing and returning to the social world after life-altering treatments remain tasks that can be accomplished best in the company of professional and family companions who can provide support and counseling along the way.

REFERENCES

Andrykowski, M. A., Brady, M. J., Greiner, C. B., Altmaier, E. M., Burish, T. G., Antin, J. H., … Henslee-Downey, P. J. (1995). "Returning to normal" following bone marrow transplantation: Outcomes, expectations and informed consent. *Bone Marrow Transplantation, 15*, 573–581.

Back, A. L., Arnold, R. M., Tulsky, J. A., Baile, W. F., & Fryer-Edwards, K. A. (2003). Teaching communication skills to medical oncology fellows. *Journal of Clinical Oncology, 21*, 2433–2436.

Bosetti, C., Garavello, W., Gallus, S., & La, V. C. (2006). Effects of smoking cessation on the risk of laryngeal cancer: An overview of published studies. *Oral Oncology, 42*, 866–872.

Cella, D. F., & Bonomi, A. E. (1995). Measuring quality of life: 1995 update. *Oncology, 9*, 47–60.

Chen, A. M., Daly, M. E., Vazquez, E., Courquin, J., Luu, Q., Donald, P. J., and Farwell, D. G. (2013). Depression among long-term survivors of head and neck cancer treated with radiation therapy. *JAMA Otolaryngology-Head & Neck Surgery, 139*, 885–889.

Cooley, C. H. (1902). *Human nature and the social order*. New York, NY: Scribners.

Derogatis, L. R., Morrow, G. R., Fetting, J., Penman, D., Piasetsky, S., Schmale, A. M., … Carnicke, C. L., Jr. (1983). The prevalence of psychiatric disorders among cancer patients. *Journal of the American Medical Association, 249*, 751–757.

Devins, G. M., Otto, K. J., Irish, J. C., & Rodin, G. M. (2010). Head and neck cancer. In J. C. Holland, W. S. Breitbart, P. B. Jacobsen, M. S. Lederberg, M. J. Loscalzo, & R. McCorkle (Eds.), *Psych-Oncology* (pp. 135–139). New York, NY: Oxford.

Duffy, S. A., Ronis, D. L., Valenstein, M., Lambert, M. T., Fowler, K. E., Gregory, L., … Terrell, J. E. (2006). A tailored smoking, alcohol, and depression intervention for head and neck cancer patients. *Cancer Epidemiology, Biomarkers & Prevention, 15*, 2203–2208.

Engel, G. L. (1977). The need for a new medical model: a challenge for biomedicine. *Science, 196*, 129–136.

Epstein, R. M. & Street, R. L., Jr. (2007). *Patient-centered communication in cancer care: Promoting healing and reducing suffering*. NIH Publication 07–6225. Bethesda, MD: National Cancer Institute.

Fisch, M. J., Titzer, M. L., Kristeller, J. L., Shen, J., Loehrer, P. J., Jung, S. H., … Einhorn, L. H. (2003). Assessment of quality of life in outpatients with advanced cancer: The accuracy of clinician estimations and the relevance of spiritual well-being—a Hoosier Oncology Group Study. *Journal of Clinical Oncology, 21*, 2754–2759.

Garg, S., Yoo, J., & Winquist, E. (2010). Nutritional support for head and neck cancer patients receiving radiotherapy: A systematic review. *Supportive Care in Cancer, 18*, 667–677.

Garland-Thomson, R. (2009). *Staring: How we look*. New York, NY: Oxford University Press.

Griffiths, G. O., Parmar, M. K., & Bailey, A. J. (1999). Physical and psychological symptoms of quality of life in the CHART randomized trial in head and neck cancer: Short-term and long-term patient reported symptoms. CHART Steering Committee. Continuous hyperfractionated accelerated radiotherapy. *British Journal of Cancer, 81*, 1196–1205.

Haisfield-Wolfe, M. E., McGuire, D. B., Soeken, K., Geiger-Brown, J., & De Forge, B. R. (2009). Prevalence and correlates of depression among patients with head and neck cancer: A systematic review of implications for research. *Oncology Nursing Forum, 36*, E107–E125.

Humphris, G., & Ozakinci, G. (2008). The AFTER intervention: A structured psychological approach to reduce fears of recurrence in patients with head and neck cancer. *British Journal of Health Psychology, 13*, 223–230.

Hurt, G. J., McQuellon, R. P., & Barrett, R. J. (1994). After treatment ends: Neutral time. *Cancer Practice, 2*, 417–420.

Institute of Medicine. (2008). *Cancer care for the whole patient: Meeting psychosocial health needs.* Washington, DC: National Academies Press.

Kilbourn, K. M., Anderson, D., Costenaro, A., Lusczakoski, K., Borrayo, E., & Raben, D. (2013). Feasibility of EASE: A psychosocial program to improve symptom management in head and neck cancer patients. *Supportive Care in Cancer, 21*, 191–200.

Knols, R., Aaronson, N. K., Uebelhart, D., Fransen, J., & Aufdemkampe, G. (2005). Physical exercise in cancer patients during and after medical treatment: A systematic review of randomized and controlled clinical trials. *Journal of Clinocal Oncology, 23*, 3830–3842.

Kotronoulas, G., Kearney, N., Maguire, R., Harrow, A., Di, D. D., Croy, S., & MacGillivray, S. (2014). What is the value of the routine use of patient-reported outcome measures toward improvement of patient outcomes, processes of care, and health service outcomes in cancer care? A systematic review of controlled trials. *Journal of Clinical Oncology, 32*, 1480–1501.

Laugsand, E. A., Sprangers, M. A., Bjordal, K., Skorpen, F., Kaasa, S., & Klepstad, P. (2010). Health care providers underestimate symptom intensities of cancer patients: A multicenter European study. *Health and Quality of Life Outcomes, 8*, 104.

Ligibel, J. (2012). Lifestyle factors in cancer survivorship. *Journal of Clinical Oncology, 30*, 3697–3704.

Luckett, T., Britton, B., Clover, K., & Rankin, N. M. (2011). Evidence for interventions to improve psychological outcomes in people with head and neck cancer: A systematic review of the literature. *Supportive Care in Cancer, 19*, 871–881.

McNeely, M. L., Parliament, M. B., Seikaly, H., Jha, N., Magee, D. J., Haykowsky, M. J., & Courneya, K. S. (2008). Effect of exercise on upper extremity pain and dysfunction in head and neck cancer survivors: A randomized controlled trial. *Cancer, 113*, 214–222.

McQuellon, R. P., Hurt, G. J., & DeChatelet, P. (1996). Psychosocial care of the patient with cancer: A model for organizing services. *Cancer Practice, 4*, 304–311.

McQuellon, R. P., Moose, D. B., Russell, G. B., Case, L. D., Greven, K., Stevens, M., & Shaw, E. G. (2002). Supportive use of megestrol acetate (Megace) with head/neck and lung cancer patients receiving radiation therapy. *International Journal of Radiation Oncology, Biology, Physics, 52*, 1180–1185.

Metcalfe, C. W., Lowe, D., & Rogers, S. N. (2014). What patients consider important: Temporal variations by early and late stage oral, oropharyngeal and laryngeal subsites. *Journal of Craniomaxillofacial Surgery, 42*, 641–647.

Meyer, A., Keszte, J., Wollbruck, D., Dietz, A., Oeken, J., Vogel, H. J., … Singer, S. (2015). Psychological distress and need for psycho-oncological support in spouses of total laryngectomised cancer patients—results for the first 3 years after surgery. *Supportive Care in Cancer, 23*,1331–1339.

Misono, S., Weiss, N. S., Fann, J. R., Redman, M., & Yueh, B. (2008). Incidence of suicide in persons with cancer. *Journal of Clinical Oncology, 26*, 4731–4738.

Moadel, A. B., Ostroff, J., & Schantz, S. P. (1998). Head and neck cancer. In J. C. Holland, W. S. Breitbart, P. B. Jacobsen, M. S. Lederberg, M. J. Loscalzo, M. J. Massie, & R. McCorkle (Eds.), *Psycho-Oncology* (pp. 314–321). New York, NY: Oxford University Press.

National Cancer Institute. (2015). Surveillance, epidemiology, and end results program. Retrieved from http://seer. cancer.gov/statfacts/html/laryn.html.

Passik, S. D., Dugan, W., McDonald, M. V., Rosenfeld, B., Theobald, D. E., & Edgerton, S. (1998). Oncologists' recognition of depression in their patients with cancer. *Journal of Clinical Oncology, 16*, 1594–1600.

Pereira da Silva, A., Feliciano, T., Vaz Freitas, S., Esteves, S., & Almeida E Sousa, C. (2015). Quality of life in patients submitted to total laryngectomy. *Journal of Voice, 29*, 382–388.

Rinkel, R. N., Verdonck-de Leeuw, I. M., van den Brakel, N., de, B. R., Eerenstein, S. E., Aaronson, N., & Leemans, C. R. (2014). Patient-reported symptom questionnaires in laryngeal cancer: Voice, speech and swallowing. *Oral Oncology, 50*, 759–764.

Rogers, L. Q., Courneya, K. S., Robbins, K. T., Malone, J., Seiz, A., Koch, L., … Nagarkar, M. (2006). Physical activity and quality of life in head and neck cancer survivors. *Supportive Care in Cancer, 14*, 1012–1019.

Singer, S., Krauss, O., Keszte, J., Siegl, G., Papsdorf, K., Severi, E., … Kortmann, R. D. (2012). Predictors of emotional distress in patients with head and neck cancer. *Head and Neck, 34*, 180–187.

Trask, P. C., Hsu, M. A., & McQuellon, R. (2009). Other paradigms: Health-related quality of life as a measure in cancer treatment: Its importance and relevance. *The Cancer Journal, 15*, 435–440.

van der Meulen, I. C., May, A. M., de Leeuw, J. R., Koole, R., Oosterom, M., Hordijk, G. J., & Ros, W. J. (2014). Long-term effect of a nurse-led psychosocial intervention on health-related quality of life in patients with head and neck cancer: A randomised controlled trial. *British Journal of Cancer, 110*, 593–601.

Wills, T. A. (1991). Social support and interpersonal relationships. In M. S. Clark (Ed.), *Prosocial behavior: Review of personality and social psychology, Vol. 12* (pp. 265–289). Newbury Park, CA: Sage Publications.

Wilson, I. B. & Cleary, P. D. (1995). Linking clinical variables with health-related quality of life. A conceptual model of patient outcomes. *Journal of the American Medical Association, 273*, 59–65.

Worden, J. W. & Weisman, A. D. (1980). Do cancer patients really want counseling? *General Hospital Psychiatry,* *2*, 100–103.

Zabora, J., BrintzenhofeSzoc, K., Curbow, B., Hooker, C., & Piantadosi, S. (2001). The prevalence of psychological distress by cancer site. *Psychooncology, 10*, 19–28.

SUGGESTED READINGS

Bar-On, D., Lazar, A., & Amir, M. (2000). Quantitative assessment of response shift in QOL research. *Social Indicators Research, 49*, 37–49.

Carlson, L. E., Angen, M., Cullum, J., Goodey, E., Koopmans, J., Lamont, L., ... Bultz, B. D. (2004). High levels of untreated distress and fatigue in cancer patients. *British Journal of Cancer, 90*, 2297–2304.

Cooley, C. H. (1902). *Human nature and the social order.* New York, NY: Scribners.

McQuellon, R. P., Hurt, G. J., & DeChatelet, P. (1996). Psychosocial care of the patient with cancer: A model for organizing services. *Cancer Practice, 4*, 304–311.

Richardson, A. E., Morton, R., & Broadbent, E. (2015). Psychological support needs of patients with head and neck cancer and their caregivers: A qualitative study. *Psychology and Health,* 1–18.

Verdonck-de Leeuw, I. M., Buffart, L. M., Heymans, M. W., Rietveld, D. H., Doornaert, P., de Bree, R., ... Langendijk, J. A. (2014). The course of health-related quality of life in head and neck cancer patients treated with chemoradiation: A prospective cohort study. *Radiotherapy and Oncology, 110*, 422–428.

Palliative Care for Patients With Laryngeal Cancer

Julia R. Brennan, BSE; Andrew J. Rosko, MD; and
Andrew G. Shuman, MD

IMPORTANCE OF PALLIATIVE CARE IN LARYNGEAL CANCER

The treatment of laryngeal cancer (LC) has advanced immensely over the past century, and clinicians now have a large armamentarium of therapeutic modalities from which they can design individualized treatment plans. Techniques for surgery, reconstruction, radiation therapy, chemotherapy, and targeted therapy have evolved, providing patients and providers with more options than ever (Shuman, Fins, & Prince, 2012). However, despite the increasing complexity of cancer treatment, there has not been a concomitant improvement in survival outcomes (Gourin et al., 2015). Patients with LC often still find themselves facing an incurable disease with significant morbidity. Many patients are ultimately forced to bear the burden of a multitude of symptoms that threaten their physical and psychological well-being (Shuman, Yang, Taylor, & Prince, 2011).

Because of the site and nature of laryngeal tumors, patients often suffer significant symptoms secondary to the tumor itself, and they often require intensive intervention to facilitate adequate nutrition, airway patency, and pain relief (Timon & Reilly, 2006). Because of the delicate nature of laryngeal anatomy, the primary tumor threatens airway obstruction, dyspnea, dysphagia, odynophagia, and aphonia, and patients with LC can have difficulty with secretion management or aspiration. More globally, patients with LC may suffer from general pain, weight loss, fatigue, or psychological issues, including altered mentation, depression, and anxiety (Price, Moore, Moynihan, & Price, 2009). As with many head and neck cancers, the diagnosis of laryngeal malignancy is often accompanied by a sense of guilt and stigma as a result of the behavioral self-blame associated with tobacco or alcohol use (Lebel et al., 2013). LC is associated with significant morbidity secondary to its critical location; therefore, patient-centered palliative management is critical for enabling patients to live with dignity and respect as they reach the end of their life (Shuman et al., 2012) (Case Study 8-1).

Friberg, J. C., & Vinney, L. A.
Laryngeal Cancer: An Interdisciplinary
Resource for Practitioners (pp. 129-141).
© 2017 Taylor and Francis Group.

CASE STUDY 8-1

PATIENT NAME: FRANK, A 65-YEAR-OLD MAN

Clinical Status: from advanced to incurable LC

Frank presented to his primary care doctor with hoarseness and throat pain and was referred to an otolaryngologist, who made the diagnosis of incurable LC. He was treated with chemotherapy and radiation. His radiation oncologist, medical oncologist, and head and neck surgeon treated his pain and other symptoms with a variety of oral and topical medications, and he recovered well.

Six months later, his pain returned because his cancer had recurred. Frank was very reluctant to have a laryngectomy but ultimately decided that he wanted to proceed with the surgery in the hope that it would cure his cancer. Surgery went well, and he worked with an SLP to regain his ability to eat and communicate.

One year later, Frank's cancer was found to have metastasized to his lungs and his neck. He was short of breath, had more secretions, and developed an ulcer in his neck next to his stoma. He was no longer able to live alone. His family was supportive but unable to take care of him. He wanted to breathe better and be without pain, but he did not want to "go into the hospital to die."

PALLIATIVE CARE AS A CONTINUUM DURING CANCER CARE

Palliative care, broadly defined, is care that strives to improve the quality of life and reduce suffering in patients with severe illness. The overarching goal of palliation is to prevent and ameliorate symptoms of the disease itself and the adverse effects of treatment. In addition to addressing the physical symptoms, palliative care also addresses the associated psychological, social, and spiritual issues that arise as a part of illness. The outcome or success of palliative therapy is not measured by its ability to cure disease or prolong life; rather, it is based on the relief of pain, suffering, and discomfort and improvement in quality of life within the contextualized and stated goals of patients and their families (World Health Organization [WHO], 2016).

In many cases, palliative care and cancer-directed therapy are inseparable. For example, early in his cancer therapy, in conjunction with his radiation and chemotherapeutic regimen, Frank received medication to treat his pain and oral and topical therapies for his mucositis (see Case Study 8-1). Even cancer-directed care can be used for palliation, because potentially incurable cancers are often treated with surgery, chemotherapy, and/or radiation to reduce symptoms and improve quality of life.

Rather than being separate entities, cancer-directed care and palliative care represent a continuum on which two major transition points fall (Boyd & Murray, 2010). Early in a treatment course, particularly for patients with presumably curable cancers, the majority of the treatment is directed at the cancer and focuses on treating the underlying malignancy. As time and the disease progress for patients whose cancers are not cured, the focus gradually transitions away from cancer-directed care and prioritizes supportive and palliative care. Another discrete transition may occur later in the disease course when it becomes clear that a patient is reaching his or her final days. At that point, the focus shifts toward terminal care and symptom management alone. As we see in the case of Frank, his course of treatment evolved from being a regimen primarily of curative intent to having an eventual focus on palliation. It is important to note, however, that even at the outset of his curative therapy, Frank was also receiving palliative therapy to address the adverse effects of his cancer and cancer treatment. Thus, palliative care should not be viewed only as an end-of-life option for patient support and/or pain management.

Despite these ambiguities, there are three prototypical situations that involve patients with LC in which the need for a palliative—as opposed to a curative—focus is most critical. These patient situations are defined in the literature as follows (Shuman et al., 2012):

1. Patients with unresectable locoregional disease, either at initial presentation or after treatment

2. Patients who are not candidates for cancer-directed therapy with curative intent because of their medical comorbidities or functional status

3. Patients who choose palliation because of individual preference and autonomy

MULTIDISCIPLINARY PALLIATIVE CARE TEAM

Palliative care encompasses a multifaceted approach to comprehensive symptom management. The breadth and scope necessitate an equally broad representation of practitioners to coordinate care. The interdisciplinary team includes physicians in otolaryngology, medical oncology, radiation oncology, *palliative medicine*, and psychiatry, among others, alongside nurses, social workers, speech-language pathologists (SLPs), nutritionists, chaplains, physical and occupational therapists, and others, all pooling their collective expertise. The group comes together to provide supportive services that best address each patient's needs (Goldstein, Genden, & Morrison, 2008).

The success of this multidisciplinary model relies on adequate communication between care providers and patients, because collaboration is critical for reaching the best decision, especially in the context of complex cases of LC (Shuman et al., 2012). Early and routine contact between multiple stakeholders is of primary importance for ensuring that a given patient receives optimal care and that his or her family receives optimal support. In addition, the nature of team-based care also promotes self-care and stress-relief among the care providers who are most prone to burnout when caring for patients with serious illness (Goldstein et al., 2008).

Although all practitioners involved in a patient's care can participate in delivering adequate palliation, there are providers with advanced training whose sole focus is dedicated to palliative care. Engaging a dedicated palliative care team early in the course of treatment can have dramatically beneficial effects. In one recent randomized study, patients assigned to early palliative care experienced better quality of life, fewer depressive symptoms, and even lived longer, despite the fact that fewer patients in the early palliative care group received aggressive end-of-life care (Ternel et al., 2010). Although these results have not been established in patients with head and neck cancer, the salient lessons still apply and offer great promise for the use of palliative care services. A palliative team may work with head and neck specialists to provide comprehensive care as a team, particularly for patients with a significant symptom burden.

IDENTIFYING GOALS OF CARE

When treating patients with LC, especially those with advanced disease, it is important to identify and discuss each patient's goals of care. These goals will be individualized and dictated by disease status, prognosis, available treatment options, and personal preferences. Establishing realistic patient-centered goals early is critical, because they are what dictate the course of treatment. After the care team members meet with the patient to identify these goals, they must then collaborate on a plan to see them through. To do so, clinicians must help the patient recognize the relative advantages, disadvantages, and limitations of the proposed treatments.

This conversation can be a difficult task for clinicians, many of whom have difficulty discussing death. Hesitancy in starting the dialogue can be a detriment to patients and their families, who strongly desire to understand the trajectory of the disease and treatment that may await.

Box 8-1
Hospice care focuses on controlling pain and other symptoms so that patients can remain as comfortable as possible when they are near the end of their life. The goal of hospice is to anticipate and manage symptoms and to neither hasten nor postpone death.

When beginning these conversations and identifying the goals of care, it is important to balance the dialogue by offering an honest assessment of what may come without creating unreasonable expectations.

If the cancer progresses, the goals of care often shift and thus require an ongoing dialogue and a steadfast, strong patient–provider relationship to facilitate the transition. In particular, during later stages of disease, patients may adjust their goals away from aggressive cancer-directed care and focus instead on end-of-life quality. It is important to note that although less than half of patients report having end-of-life discussions, such discussions are not associated with poor mental health outcomes (Wright et al., 2008). The progression of disease and timing of death in patients with LC are uncertain, and the transition to end-of-life care can be unexpected. However, the topic of terminal care need not be postponed until death is imminent. By approaching these conversations early and proactively, providers and patients can facilitate more constructive, satisfying dialogues about the goals of care. In addition, opportunities to discuss advanced directives and identify surrogate decision makers can be critically important for ensuring that the patients' autonomy is maintained and their wishes are respected (Shuman et al., 2011).

End-of-life experiences are typically improved when patients with head and neck cancer receive care outside the hospital, although exceptions do exist. Hospitalized patients invariably undergo more invasive procedures and interventions that are not always geared toward symptom control. In addition, hospital staff rotate with each shift, and this intrinsic discontinuity in care can pave the way for misunderstanding a patient's care goals. One study revealed that many hospitalized patients with LC do not have their code status properly documented and that more than half of the patients with head and neck cancer do not have family present at the time of their death (Ethunandan, Rennie, Hoffman, Morey, & Brennan, 2005). As a result, it is often in patients' best interests to avoid unnecessary hospitalization near the end of life (Shuman et al., 2012). To accomplish this goal, families need to be prepared and provided adequate support to avoid unnecessary or unwanted readmission to a hospital. However, it is important to stress that there still will be individual medical and social situations in which hospitalization is unavoidable and/or in a patient's best interest.

As cancer progresses further and a patient reaches the terminal phase of disease, enrollment in a hospice program becomes an important consideration (Box 8-1). It is critical for patients to know that hospice care can be discontinued and active treatment may resume if the patient changes his or her mind, if medical circumstances change, or if new treatments become available. Hospice care most often takes place at the patient's home, but it can also be delivered at special inpatient facilities, hospitals, and nursing homes. Qualifying for hospice care typically requires formal recognition/acceptance from the patient and his or her family and a statement from a doctor and the hospice medical director that the patient has a life expectancy of 6 months or less if the disease runs its normal course. Because there are unknowns with any predictions, hospice care can be continued if a patient lives longer than 6 months, as long as the hospice medical director or other hospice doctor recertifies the patient's condition and prognosis.

SYMPTOM MANAGEMENT

Locoregional Treatment Toxicity

Palliative care can play many roles in addressing symptoms that result from the LC itself but also in addressing the adverse sequelae of therapies during all phases of care, which is when blurring of the line between palliative and curative care arises (Goldstein et al., 2008). Radiation therapy can produce dramatically troublesome side effects in patients with head and neck cancer, and it is best for care providers to prepare themselves and their patients for these eventualities before they occur. Patients may notice only mild symptoms of dry mouth early in treatment; however, after 3 or 4 weeks of radiation therapy, most patients suffer debilitating mucositis, xerostomia, dermatitis, and soft-tissue damage to the areas around their face and neck. Anticipation, prevention, and aggressive management are the cornerstones of palliative care to provide support to patients exhibiting these treatment effects. Although some of the material presented here is discussed in earlier chapters of this book, its mention is important here, as well, to highlight the role that palliative care plays in integrating the functions of the LC care team in adopting the mission of treating the whole patient as treatment for LC is pursued and/or end-of-life decisions are made. Although palliative care physicians typically manage these treatment effects, other allied health personnel can be involved also (Table 8-1).

Mucositis

Mucositis results from inflammation and breakdown of the mucus membranes after exposure to radiation and/or chemotherapy and causes pain and difficulty eating and managing secretions. These symptoms can lead to severe malnutrition and weight loss in affected patients (Xing & Zhang, 2015). The application of topical anesthetic mouthwash has been shown to provide temporary pain relief in patients suffering from oral mucositis (Ballonoff, Chen, & Raben, 2006). Systemic opioids have also been shown to be effective in treating the pain of mucositis, and they are indicated if local treatments are insufficient (Goldstein et al., 2008). Treating the pain associated with mucositis by using topical anesthetics or analgesics is critical for promoting proper nutritional intake and improving quality of life during and after radiation therapy (Xing & Zhang, 2015). Symptoms can be exacerbated after superinfection by either *Candida* or oral bacterial flora. Using baking soda mouthwash, antifungal mouthwash, and/or nystatin (an antifungal medication) can be important for preventing the onset of these secondary infections. Mucositis can also present with substantial swelling, for which nonsteroidal anti-inflammatory agents or steroids may provide relief (Ballonoff et al., 2006).

Xerostomia

Symptoms of xerostomia (radiation-induced dry mouth) are also a common complication that results from radiation damage to salivary glands. Xerostomia may persist for several months to years after treatment, and in some cases, the effects are lifelong. Deficits in the production of saliva can be associated with difficulty eating, swallowing, speaking, and maintaining proper dental hygiene (Brosky, 2007). Palliative measures for patients who suffer xerostomia are targeted toward keeping the mouth lubricated and stimulating salivary flow. These measures include liberal hydration/humidification, the use of salivary substitutes to hydrate the mucosa, and gustatory stimulants (Goldstein et al., 2008). Parasympathomimetic agents such as pilocarpine and cevimeline can also improve a patient's symptoms by reducing dryness and mitigating oral discomfort, but they are not without adverse effects (Fogh & Yom, 2014; Shiboski, Hodgson, Ship, & Schiødt, 2007). It is recommended that all patients with head and neck cancer visit a dentist before starting radiation treatment and receive dental care throughout the course of and subsequent to therapy. Radiation-induced damage to the salivary glands increases the risk of *dental caries* (tooth decay), which

TABLE 8-1

APPROACHES TO MANAGING
LARYNGEAL CANCER SYMPTOMS AND SIDE EFFECTS

SYMPTOM	APPROACHES TO MANAGEMENT
Inflammation of the mouth after radiation (mucositis)	Anesthetic mouthwash for pain
	Analgesic medications for pain
	Baking soda or antifungal mouthwash for prevention of infection
	Anti-inflammatory medications for swelling
Dry mouth after radiation (xerostomia)	Salivary substitutes or stimulants
	Hydration and lubrication
	Dental consultation for prevention of cavities
Skin reactions after radiation (dermatitis)	Moisturizer before radiation
	Ointments after radiation
	Loose-fitting clothing around the neck and affected area
Swallowing difficulties (dysphagia and odynophagia)	Short-term high-dose corticosteroids for nausea and appetite loss
	Analgesic medications for pain
	Artificial nutrition and hydration
Communication difficulties	Alternative communication methods (see Chapter 5)
	Speech and language pathology consultations
Pain	Analgesic medications for pain from tissue damage
	Anticonvulsants, antidepressants, or local anesthetics for pain from nerve damage
	Complementary and alternative pain management (e.g., massage, acupuncture)
Psychiatric needs	Early psychiatric consultation (even before starting therapy)
	Antidepressants and psychotherapy for depression; support groups for anxiety

requires fluoride therapy, preventive maintenance, and judicious interventions (Ballonoff et al., 2006).

Skin Reactions

Patients with LC may experience various degrees of dermatitis and soft-tissue damage to the skin of their head and neck within the treatment field. This damage ensues because radiation inadvertently targets the rapidly dividing cells of the epidermis, sebaceous (oil) glands, and hair follicles, which results in an inflammatory response to tissue injury (Fogh & Yom, 2014). The exposed field may become edematous before ultimately blistering, ulcerating, and sloughing (Goldstein et al., 2008). Moisturizer can be applied prophylactically to prevent severe reactions from occurring. Unscented topical ointments, aloe, or corticosteroid cream can also be helpful for lower-grade dermatitis, but patients should avoid products that contain alcohol, menthol, or perfume. Patients should also avoid trauma and further irritation by wearing loose-fitting clothing around the neck and affected area, and itching in the area should be minimized (Fogh & Yom, 2014). Longstanding induration (hardening of normally soft tissue), irritation, lymphedema, and stiffness require chronic range-of-motion exercise and massage.

Airway Management

Airway management presents as a common issue among patients with LC (refer to Chapter 4 for additional detailed information regarding airway and respiratory challenges for patients with LC). These challenges can be managed by physicians, respiratory therapists, and (at times) SLPs. Issues with the airway may arise from the tumor itself or as a consequence of the therapy administered (Goldstein et al., 2008). Studies in LC care in elderly patients have found that higher-quality patient-centered care is associated with a reduced incidence of airway and swallowing impairment after treatment. In these cases, quality indicators are defined by evidence-based standards of care defined by the National Comprehensive Cancer Network (NCCN) and by literature on end-of-life care (Gourin et al., 2015). Particularly for patients with recurrent or incurable disease, the possibility of airway compromise is anticipated ideally well in advance so that patients and their families and providers can make decisions regarding airway management long before any interventions need to be put into emergent action. This type of proactive dialogue with patients and their surrogate decision makers can be critical for avoiding situations in which decision making is forced by clinical emergencies that compromise patients' ability to exercise their autonomy (Shuman et al., 2012). Given the difficulties inherent in emergent airway interventions, these discussions can be used by clinicians to consider and clarify the goals of care. They can also be used as a means to introduce other more supportive measures to proactively address airway emergencies as a means of avoiding the consequences that come with achieving definitive airway control (Shuman et al., 2013). Studies have shown that critically ill patients can benefit from electing to have a tracheotomy performed proactively, which likely results in decreased risk of death (Correia, Sousa, Pinto, & Barros, 2014). The prolongation of life alongside the palliative improvements in symptom management—particularly shortness of breath—may outweigh the risks of the procedure and logistic hurdles of managing a tracheostomy tube and make it a viable option for many patients with LC. However, other patients, including those with progressive terminal disease, may reasonably choose to forego airway interventions and opt to treat symptoms expectantly.

Dysphagia and Odynophagia

Swallowing difficulties in patients with LC can present as dysphagia or odynophagia and often manifest with reduced nutritional intake and weight loss (refer to Chapter 6 for additional information about management of dysphagia for patients with LC). In conjunction with palliative care specialists, both dietitians and SLPs play significant roles in the management of these issues. This complication has been shown to have significant implications on quality of life in patients with cancer (Terrell et al., 2004). Short-term high-dose corticosteroids are frequently administered to reduce the incidence of anorexia, nausea, and other symptoms, but the patient may ultimately require artificial hydration and nutritional support (Shuman et al., 2012). Systemic opioids can also be effective in patients with severe odynophagia, for whom pain relief facilitates their ability to swallow (Goldstein et al., 2008). Palliation of severe pain for patients with cancer—particularly in the context of terminal disease—is clearly recognized as a setting in which the risk of opioid addiction is drastically superseded by the indication for symptom control (Krashin, Murinova, Jumelle, & Ballantyne, 2015). In addition, aggressive humidification can inhibit desiccation, crusting, and obstruction (Shuman et al., 2012).

Artificial nutrition and hydration are commonly administered through a gastrostomy tube and ensure that patients receive sufficient hydration and nutrition, especially during the healing process. If nutritional access is necessary for only a short period, such as during chemoradiation, then temporary nasogastric access can be extremely useful; it prevents an unnecessary surgical procedure and can be placed in clinic. The preferred method of gastric feeding is bolus feeding, which permits large quantities of nutrients to be delivered in short regular intervals and gives patients the freedom to go about their day without the inconvenience of a pump. Consultation with a dietitian can ensure that patients receive the necessary amount of calories, protein, and water and avoid complications related to tube feeding (Goldstein et al., 2008).

Communication

Because of its anatomic location, LC is intrinsically linked to communication. Oftentimes, patients must rely on inventive methods of communication to interact with their family, friends, and providers, without which these patients would suffer even greater psychological and psychosocial harm from their conditions. It is the responsibility of the caregivers to do their part to ensure that the patient's voice is being heard, even when the limitations of disease make it a physical impossibility (Shuman et al., 2012). For patients with head and neck cancer, decision making requires patient-centric input regarding personal considerations of values, quality of life, physiological function, and attitudes toward aggressive symptom management (Shuman et al., 2013). Using open and inventive communication, decisions are made not in isolation but, rather, in an environment in which there is honest discussion about prognosis, possible outcomes, and the options that are and are not available going forward (Ethunandan et al., 2005). Speech-language pathologists are integral to these discussions in terms of offering support and education for patients and their families.

As discussed in Chapter 5, the choice of communication method after treatment for LC is personal in its own right and may depend on a given patient's anatomy, cognitive ability, and physical capacity. Devices such as one-way speaking valves, electrolarynxes, computer-driven communication software, and alternative speaking techniques can be useful to some patients, whereas others might opt for a paper and pencil to use for communication (Shuman et al., 2012). In the case of Frank, his laryngectomy affected his capacity to communicate, but he was ultimately able to regain his ability to speak fluently after working with an SLP. His case study highlights another important facet of the multidisciplinary palliative care team at work; patients with LC benefit from early and regular collaboration with SLPs, particularly those who specialize in the care of patients with a head or neck malignancy (Goldstein et al., 2008).

Pain

Patients with LC almost universally experience pain at some point in their disease-management process. In early-stage cancers, pain can be managed fairly routinely and for intermittent periods of time. In later stages of LC, pain can be constant, which makes pain management central to maintaining quality of life. Beyond this, the top priority for patients and providers is a painless and comfortable death, free of distressing symptoms (Ethunandan et al., 2005).

Pain with LC can be *nociceptive* and arise from the tumor itself as it relates to the destruction of tissue, or it can be neuropathic and arise from damage to the surrounding nerve fibers. It can also arise as an adverse effect of one or more therapeutic modalities being used to treat the cancer. Nociceptive pain responds to analgesia and is treated with either peripherally active nonsteroidal anti-inflammatory drugs or centrally acting opioid medications (Binczak et al., 2014). Systemic opioid administration can be limited by the adverse effects it elicits, including nausea, dysphoria, delirium, lethargy, and respiratory depression. In patients with head and neck cancer especially, these complications can make it difficult to maintain therapeutic medication levels (Miyazaki, Satou, Ohno, Yoshida, & Nishimura, 2014). Neuropathic pain is often treated with anticonvulsants, tricyclic antidepressants, local anesthetics, and other medications (Lussier, Huskey, & Portenoy, 2004).

The available route of administration of pharmaceuticals is often dictated by the patient's swallowing function. In patients with feeding tubes, delayed-release enteral (by mouth) formulations are not possible. Transdermal fentanyl administration is an effective alternative for long-acting pain control (Xing & Zhang, 2015). Liquid morphine has also been successful in controlling pain and provides another suitable option for patients with head and neck cancer (Olsen & Creagan,

1991). Finally, the subcutaneous drug-administration route has typically been the standard of practice for terminally ill patients and may be presented as an earlier option for patients with head and neck cancer, given their limitations (Ethunandan et al., 2005).

Complementary and alternative options for pain control are also available, but their uses are associated with various results. These options include massage for muscle pain, acupuncture for acute or postoperative pain, and herbal supplements for generalized pain management. Some patients may find these tools to be useful (Leong, Smith, & Rowland-Seymour, 2015).

The NCCN has a guideline that suggests that a patient's palliative care needs be assessed early and continually and that patients with complicated needs be referred to a palliative care specialist (Yoshimoto et al., 2015). The NCCN guidelines, alongside an algorithm developed by the WHO, provide practitioners and patients with the core principles of cancer pain management. They also address the vast range of complexities and comorbidities facing these patients with cancer and provide information on dosing, drug combinations, and adverse effects of opioids, nonopioid analgesics, and adjuvant analgesics (Swarm et al., 2013).

Depression

The process of undergoing diagnosis and treatment of LC can be exceedingly taxing on a patient, which can result in a compromised quality of life. The larynx is a complex structure with a critical function for activities of daily living, and, as such, damage to the area can have significant emotional and social effects (Murphy, Ridner, Wells, & Dietrich, 2007). In addition, patients with head and neck cancer have been found to have a high incidence of pre-existing comorbid psychiatric disease and depressive symptoms, which, combined with the associations head and neck cancer has with tobacco and alcohol abuse, lack of social support, and low socioeconomic status, predisposes this population of patients to increased incidences of depressive symptoms (Chan et al., 2011). Studies have shown quality of life in patients with head and neck cancer to be profoundly affected by treatment-related side effects and disease-specific problems but also that management and resolution of these problems lead to long-term normalization of reported quality of life (Hammerlid & Taft, 2001).

Of particular importance are the rates of depression in this population undergoing radiation therapy. Depression is reported to be prevalent in approximately half of the patients with head and neck cancer before treatment with radiation, and this number climbs even higher during the course of the therapy (Chen et al., 2009). In addition, researchers found that rates of suicide in patients with LC are significantly higher than those in the general population and, notably, higher than those in most populations of patients with other types of cancer (Misono, Weiss, Fann, Redman, & Yueh, 2008). These rates are thought to be results of the disproportionate impact this cancer has on quality of life and the fact that substance abuse is common (Hammerlid & Taft, 2001; Zeller, 2006).

Prophylactic medical treatment with a selective serotonin-reuptake inhibitor has been shown to reduce the risk of depression in patients with head and neck cancer and offer significant improvements in reported quality of life (Lydiatt, Bessette, Schmid, Sayles, & Burke, 2013). Cognitive behavioral therapy (discussed more in Chapter 7) and other antidepressants are also effective interventions for depressive symptoms, and they can be similarly useful in treating comorbid smoking and problem drinking disorders as well (Duffy et al., 2006). However, it is worth noting that many of these same patients will be suffering from xerostomia, and these patients are often advised against using tricyclic antidepressants because of their anticholinergic potentiation of the side effects of dry mouth (Goldstein et al., 2008). Early consultation with a psychiatrist, counselor, and/or relevant clergy can be instrumental in addressing these concerns and, ultimately, can provide a considerable benefit to the complete palliative care regimen (Shapiro & Kornfeld, 1987). In addition to this early consult, every patient should be routinely screened for depression and other psychiatric needs, because mental well-being is a critical component of head and neck cancer care.

Anxiety

Patients with head and neck malignancy are at high risk for both locoregional recurrence and metastatic spread, which can contribute to a near-constant sense of anxiety related to concerns of relapse (Goldstein et al., 2008). Although pharmacological antianxiety treatment may be indicated for some patients, studies have found that head and neck cancer support groups can provide significant improvements in rates of reported emotional distress and in other quality-of-life domains (Vakharia, Ali, & Wang, 2007). Clinicians can play an important role by merely starting this conversation and connecting their patients with these support groups (Goldstein et al., 2008). In addition, a patient's pre-existing familial and social support groups can be valuable partners in maintaining the patient's well-being, and these groups can be an important resource for the palliative care team.

Guilt and Self-Blame

The epidemiological links between tobacco and alcohol use and head and neck cancers have been well established, and LC is no exception. Rates of LC are highest among those who have had the longest duration of use and the greatest consumption of tobacco and alcohol, and the use of both substances increases the risk even more (Haws & Haws, 2014). Some patients may blame themselves for the role their behaviors may have had in their diagnosis, while others may experience feelings of guilt about the toll that the illness takes on their family and caregivers (Goldstein et al., 2008). Patients who engage in greater degrees of self-blame end up facing more negative pretreatment illness perceptions. Studies have suggested that this guilt is linked to not only a lesser quality of life but also an increased risk of poor adjustment to cancer therapy (Christensen et al., 1999).

Patients may feel stigmatized by their behaviors, and they may be reluctant to disclose their former or ongoing use of tobacco or alcohol, which illustrates a lost opportunity for intervention on the part of the provider to assist in a patient's process of quitting or maintaining abstinence (Simmons et al., 2009). The medical team can avoid this loss by proactively examining these issues and restructuring the patient's perception of the illness with the appropriately framed information.

Studies have found that approximately one-third of patients with lung and head and neck cancers continue to smoke after receiving their diagnosis (Burris, Studts, DeRosa, & Ostroff, 2015). Patients who attribute their cancer to past substance abuse exhibit a lower likelihood of smoking but only if they also understand their future cancer-related outcomes to be contingent on smoking cessation (Christensen et al., 1999). By taking a more active role in recognizing and addressing the emotional well-being of the patient, members of the LC care team (e.g., palliative physicians, counselors, psychiatrists) can facilitate a more empowered awareness and emphasize the importance of self-care in this vulnerable population (Scharloo et al., 2005).

Body Image

LC strips its victims of a vital component of their identity and, in doing so, poses distinctly complex physiological and psychological issues for patients and providers alike (Shuman et al., 2012). Changes in body appearance and self-perception are extremely common, and they can be debilitating. Studies have linked dissatisfaction with body image and greater symptom severity with negative changes in the frequency with which a patient with LC speaks after treatment relative to before treatment (Chen et al., 2015), which represents yet another barrier to communication for these patients in whom functional deficits may already be present.

Head and neck cancer can be quite disfiguring. Similarly, because of the substantial impact this cancer has on swallowing and nutrition, weight loss and *cachexia* (decreased cell body mass caused by cancer) can have a negative psychological impact as well (Goldstein et al., 2008). The malignancy itself, the treatment regimen, and the side effects all contribute to this detrimental decrease in physical functioning and body image. The accumulation of all of these factors contributes to globally decreased quality of life among patients with head and neck cancer (Hammerlid & Taft, 2001).

Disfigurement of the head and neck, physiological impairments, and general loss of self-esteem can be extremely damaging to a patient's therapeutic progress, and it is the responsibility of the care team to address these issues. A psychiatrist and/or psychosocial oncology counselor/specialist can be an instrumental addition to the care team for assisting patients in managing what might be traumatic changes. Group support provides another opportunity for addressing these issues in an effective empathetic setting (Callahan, 2004) and is another situation in which the importance of the palliative care team in confronting these very real, multifaceted issues in this population of patients with cancer is illustrated.

CONCLUSION

Palliation of symptoms is critically important when caring for patients with LC regardless of their age or tumor stage. The effects of the cancer itself and the therapies deployed to treat the disease impose a significant burden on patients. The anatomic location and delicate structures found there make symptoms unique and challenging relative to those in other sites, and optimal care requires a multidisciplinary approach. Palliative care is a continuum that encompasses care for the patient from diagnosis through end-of-life care and focuses more on symptoms and disease burden rather than survival. In addition, early engagement of a palliative care team can be beneficial and results in vast improvements in quality of life. Thus, it is likely that all members of the LC care team will need to assist with palliation over the course of a patient's disease and life trajectory.

REFERENCES

Ballonoff, A., Chen, C., & Raben, D. (2006). Current radiation therapy management issues in oral cavity cancer. *Otolaryngologic Clinics of North America, 39,* 365–380.

Binczak, M., Navez, M., Perrichon, C., Blanchard, D., Bollet, M., Calmels, P., ... SFORL Work Group. (2014). Management of somatic pain induced by head-and-neck cancer treatment: Definition and assessment. Guidelines of the French Oto-Rhino-Laryngology-Head and Neck Surgery Society (SFORL). *European Annals of Otorhinolaryngology, Head and Neck Diseases, 131,* 243–247.

Boyd, K., & Murray, S. A. (2010). Recognising and managing key transitions in end of life care. *British Medical Journal, 341,* c4863.

Brosky, M. E. (2007). The role of saliva in oral health: Strategies for prevention and management of xerostomia. *Journal of Supportive Oncology, 5,* 215–225.

Burris, J. L., Studts, J. L., DeRosa, A. P., & Ostroff, J. S. (2015). Systematic review of tobacco use after lung or head/neck cancer diagnosis: Results and recommendations for future research. *Cancer Epidemiology, Biomarkers & Prevention, 24,* 1450–1461.

Callahan, C. (2004). Facial disfigurement and sense of self in head and neck cancer. *Social Work in Health Care, 40,* 73–87.

Chan, J. Y. K., Lua, L. L., Starmer, H. H., Sun, D. Q., Rosenblatt, E. S., & Gourin, C. G. (2011). The relationship between depressive symptoms and initial quality of life and function in head and neck cancer. *The Laryngoscope, 121,* 1212–1218.

Chen, A. M., Jennelle, R. L. S., Grady, V., Tovar, A., Bowen, K., Simonin, P., ... Vijayakumar, S. (2009). Prospective study of psychosocial distress among patients undergoing radiotherapy for head and neck cancer. *International Journal of Radiation Oncology, Biology, Physics, 73,* 187–193.

Chen, S. C., Yu, P. J., Hong, M. Y., Chen, M. H., Chu, P. Y., Chen, Y. J., ... Lai, Y. H. (2015). Communication dysfunction, body image, and symptom severity in postoperative head and neck cancer patients: Factors associated with the amount of speaking after treatment. *Supportive Care in Cancer, 23,* 2375–2382.

Christensen, A. J., Moran, P. J., Ehlers, S. L., Raichle, K., Karnell, L., & Funk, G. (1999). Smoking and drinking behavior in patients with head and neck cancer: Effects of behavioral self-blame and perceived control. *Journal of Behavioral Medicine, 22,* 407–418.

Correia, I. A. M., Sousa, V., Pinto, L. M., & Barros, E. (2014). Impact of early elective tracheotomy in critically ill patients. *Brazilian Journal of Otorhinolaryngology, 80,* 428–434.

Duffy, S. A., Ronis, D. L., Valenstein, M., Lambert, M. T., Fowler, K. E., Gregory, L., … Terrell, J. E. (2006). A tailored smoking, alcohol, and depression intervention for head and neck cancer patients. *Cancer Epidemiology, Biomarkers & Prevention, 15*, 2203–2208.

Ethunandan, M., Rennie, A., Hoffman, G., Morey, P. J., & Brennan, P. A. (2005). Quality of dying in head and neck cancer patients: A retrospective analysis of potential indicators of care. *Oral Surgery, Oral Medicine, Oral Pathology, Oral Radiology, and Endodontics, 100*, 147–152.

Fogh, S., & Yom, S. S. (2014). Symptom management during the radiation oncology treatment course: A practical guide for the oncology clinician. *Seminars in Oncology, 41*, 764–775.

Goldstein, N. E., Genden, E., & Morrison, R. (2008). Palliative care for patients with head and neck cancer: "I would like a quick return to a normal lifestyle." *Journal of the American Medical Association, 299*, 1818–1825.

Gourin, C. G., Starmer, H. M., Herbert, R. J., Frick, K. D., Forastiere, A. A., Quon, H., … Dy, S. M. (2015). Quality of care and short- and long-term outcomes of laryngeal cancer care in the elderly. *The Laryngoscope, 125*, 2323–2329.

Hammerlid, E., & Taft, C. (2001). Health-related quality of life in long-term head and neck cancer survivors: A comparison with general population norms. *British Journal of Cancer, 84*, 149–156.

Haws, L., & Haws, B. T. (2014). Aerodigestive cancers: Laryngeal cancer. *Family Practice Essentials, 424*, 26–31.

Krashin, D., Murinova, N., Jumelle, P., & Ballantyne, J. (2015). Opioid risk assessment in palliative medicine. *Expert Opinion on Drug Safety, 14*, 1023–1033.

Lebel, S., Feldstain, A., McCallum, M., Beattie, S., Irish, J., Bezjak, A., & Devins, G. M. (2013). Do behavioural self-blame and stigma predict positive health changes in survivors of lung or head and neck cancers? *Psychology & Health, 28*, 1066–1081.

Leong, M., Smith, T. J., & Rowland-Seymour, A. (2015). Complementary and integrative medicine for older adults in palliative care. *Clinics in Geriatric Medicine, 31*, 177–191.

Lussier, D., Huskey, A. G., & Portenoy, R. K. (2004). Adjuvant analgesics in cancer pain management. *The Oncologist, 9*, 571–591.

Lydiatt, W. M., Bessette, D., Schmid, K. K., Sayles, H., & Burke, W. J. (2013). Prevention of depression with escitalopram in patients undergoing treatment for head and neck cancer: Randomized, double-blind, placebo-controlled clinical trial. *JAMA Otolaryngology–Head & Neck Surgery, 139*, 678–686.

Misono, S., Weiss, N. S., Fann, J. R., Redman, M., & Yueh, B. (2008). Incidence of suicide in persons with cancer. *Journal of Clinical Oncology, 26*, 4731–4738.

Miyazaki, T., Satou, S., Ohno, T., Yoshida, A., & Nishimura, K. (2014). Topical morphine gel for pain management in head and neck cancer patients. *Auris, Nasus, Larynx, 41*, 496–498.

Murphy, B. A., Ridner, S., Wells, N., & Dietrich, M. (2007). Quality of life research in head and neck cancer: A review of the current state of the science. *Critical Reviews in Oncology/Hematology, 62*, 251–267.

Olsen, K. D., & Creagan, E. T. (1991). Pain management in advanced carcinoma of the head and neck. *American Journal of Otolaryngology, 12*, 154–160.

Price, K. A. R., Moore, E. J., Moynihan, T., & Price, D. L. (2009). Symptoms and terminal course of patients who died of head and neck cancer. *Journal of Palliative Medicine, 12*, 117–118.

Scharloo, M., Baatenburg de Jong, R. J., Langeveld, T. P. M., van Velzen-Verkaik, E., Doorn-op den Akker, M. M., & Kaptein, A. A. (2005). Quality of life and illness perceptions in patients with recently diagnosed head and neck cancer. *Head & Neck, 27*, 857–863.

Shapiro, P. A., & Kornfeld, D. S. (1987). Psychiatric aspects of head and neck cancer surgery. *Psychiatric Clinics of North America, 10*, 87–100.

Shiboski, C. H., Hodgson, T. A., Ship, J. A., & Schiødt, M. (2007). Management of salivary hypofunction during and after radiotherapy. *Oral Surgery, Oral Medicine, Oral Pathology, Oral Radiology, and Endodontics, 103*, S66. e1-S66.e19.

Shuman, A. G., Fins, J. J., & Prince, M. E. (2012). Improving end-of-life care for head and neck cancer patients. *Expert Review of Anticancer Therapy, 12*, 335–343.

Shuman, A. G., McCabe, M. S., Fins, J. J., Kraus, D. H., Shah, J. P., & Patel, S. G. (2013). Clinical ethics consultation in patients with head and neck cancer. *Head & Neck, 35*, 1647–1651.

Shuman, A. G., Yang, Y., Taylor, J. M. G., & Prince, M. E. (2011). End-of-life care among head and neck cancer patients. *Otolaryngology–Head and Neck Surgery, 144*, 733–739.

Simmons, V. N., Litvin, E. B., Patel, R. D., Jacobsen, P. B., McCaffrey, J. C., Bepler, G., … Brandon, T. H. (2009). Patient-provider communication and perspectives on smoking cessation and relapse in the oncology setting. *Patient Education and Counseling, 77*, 398–403.

Swarm, R. A., Abernethy, A. P., Anghelescu, D. L., Benedetti, C., Buga, S., Cleeland, C., … National Comprehensive Cancer Network. (2013). Adult cancer pain. *Journal of the National Comprehensive Cancer Network, 11*, 992–1022.

Ternel, J. S., Greer, J. A., Muzikansky, A., Gallagher, E. R., Admane, S., Jackson, V. A., … Lynch, T. J. (2010). Early palliative care for patients with metastatic non-small-cell lung cancer. *New England Journal of Medicine, 363*, 733–742.

Terrell, J. E., Ronis, D. L., Fowler, K. E., Bradford, C. R., Chepeha, D. B., Prince, M. E., … Duffy, S. A. (2004). Clinical predictors of quality of life in patients with head and neck cancer. *Archives of Otolaryngology–Head & Neck Surgery, 130*, 401–408.

Timon, C., & Reilly, K. (2006). Head and neck mucosal squamous cell carcinoma: Results of palliative management. *Journal of Laryngology and Otology, 120*, 389–392.

Vakharia, K. T., Ali, M. J., & Wang, S. J. (2007). Quality-of-life impact of participation in a head and neck cancer support group. *Otolaryngology–Head and Neck Surgery, 136*, 405–410.

World Health Organization. (2016). Palliative care is an essential part of cancer control. Retrieved from http://www.who.int/cancer/palliative/en/.

Wright, A. A., Zhang, B., Ray, A., Mack, J. W., Trice, E., Balboni, T., … Prigerson, H. G. (2008). Associations between end-of-life discussions, patient mental health, medical care near death, and caregiver bereavement adjustment. *Journal of the American Medical Association, 300*, 1665–1673.

Xing, S.-Z., & Zhang, Y. (2015). Efficacy and safety of transdermal fentanyl for the treatment of oral mucositis pain caused by chemoradiotherapy in patients with esophageal squamous cell carcinoma. *Supportive Care in Cancer, 23*, 753–759.

Yoshimoto, T., Tomiyasu, S., Saeki, T., Tamaki, T., Hashizume, T., Murakami, M., … Symptom Control Research Group (SCORE-G). (2015). How do hospital palliative care teams use the WHO guidelines to manage unrelieved cancer pain? A 1-year, multicenter audit in Japan. *American Journal of Hospice & Palliative Care, pii*, 1049909115608810.

Zeller, J. L. (2006). High suicide risk found for patients with head and neck cancer. *Journal of the American Medical Association, 296*, 1716–1717.

Glossary

adjuvant therapy: Therapy given after a primary treatment for cancer in an effort to make the primary treatment more effective and prevent cancer recurrence.

alaryngeal speech: Postlaryngectomy communication, including speech via an electrolarynx, and tracheoesophageal and esophageal speech.

anastomosis stricture: Development of scar tissue at the junction of the neopharynx and cervical esophagus that may narrow the esophageal opening and lead to dysphagia.

artificial larynx: Mechanical or electronic device that a laryngectomee can use as a sound source for speech.

aspiration: When foreign materials, such as food or liquids, enter the lungs by way of the trachea.

aspiration pneumonia: Bacterial infection caused by the intrusion of food/liquid into the lungs.

augmentative/alternative communication: Nonoral communication.

bedside swallow evaluation (BSE): Observation of swallowing function, conducted without imaging technology, to determine whether there are signs or symptoms of dysphagia.

benign: Growth that is not cancerous and does not spread to other areas of the body; a benign tumor may still be dangerous depending on its area of origin and effect on function.

biopsy: Surgical procedure to remove live tissue from the body so that it can be examined in a laboratory for signs of disease, such as cancer.

bolus: Small mass of chewed food and saliva.

cachexia: Malnutrition and skeletal muscle loss that is associated with chronic diseases, such as cancer.

chemoradiation: Cancer treatment that combines chemotherapy and radiation.

chemotherapy: Drug treatment for cancer.

clinical psychologist: Mental health professional who provides services including assessment and counseling to patients with psychological disorders.

computed tomography (CT): Type of diagnostic imaging that uses ionizing radiation (i.e., X-ray technology) to compile views of the body structures from many different angles that may be examined together as a three-dimensional image; often used to determine whether cancer is present in the head, neck, abdomen, or spine.

corticosteroid: Steroid hormone that is used to treat various conditions, including stress responses and inflammation.

cuff: Internal balloon that surrounds the outer body of a tracheostomy tube and prevents external ventilation from leaking into the upper airway.

debulking: Partial surgical removal of a tumor, performed when complete surgical excision is impossible, in an effort to facilitate improved chemotherapy and radiation outcomes.

decannulation button (or plug): Used to occlude the opening of the tracheostomy tube and ensure that respiration through the upper airway is tolerated before decannulation.

diagnostic radiologist: Physician who is trained to use imaging techniques as part of the assessment process to diagnose a variety of diseases, including laryngeal cancer.

dietitian: Allied health professional who assesses the adequacy of patients' nutritional requirements and provides support to ensure that they are met.

Friberg, J. C., & Vinney, L. A.
Laryngeal Cancer: An Interdisciplinary Resource for Practitioners (pp. 143-148).
© 2017 Taylor and Francis Group.

direct (operative) laryngoscopy: Procedure performed in the hospital (with the patient under general anesthesia) in which an illuminated tube is placed into the throat of a patient lying supine to visualize the larynx closely, particularly during surgery or biopsy.

dysgeusia: Dysfunction or distortion of taste sensation.

dysphagia: Disordered or difficulty swallowing.

dyspnea: Difficulty breathing (i.e., shortness of breath).

electrolarynx: Battery-operated device that produces mechanical vibration and can be used as an artificial sound source for alaryngeal speech after laryngectomy.

endoscope: Small lighted tube used to look inside a body cavity or organ, such as the larynx, during a procedure termed endoscopy.

enteral nutrition: Typically refers to the delivery of nutrition to the gastrointestinal tract via tube feedings, as opposed to parenteral nutrition, which is delivered intravenously.

epiglottic inversion: Downward movement of the epiglottis over the laryngeal vestibule during swallowing.

epiglottis: Elastic cartilage that attaches to the base of the tongue and sits directly above the entrance of the laryngeal vestibule.

erythema: Tissue irritation that results in redness.

esophageal dilation: Procedure that facilitates improved swallow function by stretching a narrowed area of the esophagus.

esophageal speech: Form of alaryngeal communication that involves vibrating the upper esophagus and lower pharynx after air is drawn into the esophagus through the mouth.

esophagus: Muscular tube that carries food, saliva, and liquid from the mouth to the stomach.

extrinsic (alaryngeal) method for communication: Communication that relies on an external source, placed in the oral cavity or the tissues of the neck, to generate sound; the most frequently used extrinsic method of communication is the electrolarynx.

fiberoptic endoscopic evaluation of swallowing (FEES): Examination of the swallowing of food or liquids, mixed with food coloring, by way of a flexible endoscope that is passed into a patient's nose and positioned in the pharynx over the larynx and upper esophagus.

fibrosis (radiation induced): Formation of excessive stiff connective tissue as a side effect of exposure to radiation treatment.

flexible fiberoptic laryngoscopy: Examination (sometimes called a nasolaryngoscopy) in which a small flexible endoscope is guided through the nose and into the pharynx to view vocal fold function from above while the patient is awake and sitting down.

foam filter (or heat and moisture exchange) cassette: Contained within the housing of a heat and moisture exchange system and placed over a stoma to allow for the humidification of inhaled air in those who breathe by way of the neck as a result of tracheotomy or laryngectomy.

gastroenterologist: Physician who specializes in treating disorders and dysfunction of the gastrointestinal tract.

gastrostomy (gastric) feeding tube (G-tube): Feeding tube inserted directly into the stomach.

glossectomy: Surgical removal of a portion of or the entire tongue.

glottic/subglottic stenosis: Narrowing at or below the glottis, often as a result of the formation of excess tissue, which may result in compromised respiration.

glottis/glottic: Space between the vocal folds visible when the vocal folds are apart (abducted). The term glottic is used to describe the location of lesions and/or food material in this region.

head and neck (HN) cancer: Cancer that affects the structures of the head and/or neck.

health-related quality of life (HR-QOL): Multidimensional concept concerned with how a person's health status affects his or her quality of life across physical, mental, emotional, and social domains.

heat and moisture exchange system (HME): System (worn over a stoma) that consists of a housing and foam filter cassette and allows for the humidification of inhaled air in those who breathe by way of the neck as a result of tracheotomy or laryngectomy.

hemilaryngectomy: Type of partial laryngectomy in which half of the larynx is removed (also called vertical partial laryngectomy).

hyolaryngeal excursion: Elevation and anterior movement of the larynx that facilitates airway protection and bolus movement during swallowing.

induction chemotherapy: First-line chemotherapy treatment (i.e., when chemotherapy is administered before another treatment such as surgery or radiation).

inner cannula: Internal portion of a tracheostomy tube that fits inside the outer cannula and functions to keep the airway patent.

insufflation: Act of drawing air into a body cavity (e.g., esophageal insufflation facilitates esophageal speech by making air available for vibration of the pharyngoesophageal segment).

intrinsic (alaryngeal) method for communication: Communication after laryngectomy that involves using anatomical body structures, such as the esophagus, as a sound source.

lary button: Silicone button that maintains the opening of a stoma by preventing any narrowing or stenosis; it may also be used as the outer housing of a heat and moisture exchange system or as an attachment site for a speaking valve.

laryngeal cancer (LC): Type of head and neck cancer that occurs when cancerous cells or tumors grow in the larynx.

laryngeal preservation: Treatment methods for laryngeal cancer that seek to avoid removal of the larynx (laryngectomy) to retain intact communication and respiratory functions.

laryngectomee: Person who has had all, or part, of his or her larynx removed.

laryngectomy: Removal of part or all of the larynx. Types of laryngectomy procedures include total laryngectomy, hemilaryngectomy, partial laryngectomy, salvage partial laryngectomy, salvage total laryngectomy, supraglottic laryngectomy, total laryngectomy.

larynx: Small cartilaginous structure that houses the vocal folds and is located between the third and sixth cervical vertebrae in adult humans.

lymph nodes: Glands of the lymphatic system that filter harmful substances and fight off infection carried by lymphatic fluid circulated throughout the body; information about the extent to which cancer has spread to nodes nearby the primary cancer site, or distant to it, factors into determination of cancer staging.

lymphadenopathy: Swollen or enlarged lymph nodes, sometimes caused by bacterial or viral infection or cancer.

lymphedema: Collection of lymph fluid that leads to swelling, often caused by a blockage in the lymphatic system that prevents the fluid from draining, and commonly results from removal of or damage to lymph nodes as part of cancer treatment(s).

magnetic resonance imaging (MRI): Type of diagnostic imaging that uses radiowaves and magnets, rather than ionizing radiation, to capture a three-dimensional image of internal tissues, joints, and ligaments.

malignant tumor: Cancerous growth that has the ability to metastasize to other parts of the body.

medical oncologist: Physician who specializes in diagnosing and/or treating cancer, most often with the use of chemotherapy.

metastasis: Progression and spread of cancerous cells from the site of origin to other parts of the body, typically through the blood or lymph system.

modified barium swallow study: *See* videofluoroscopic swallowing study (VFSS).

mucociliary lavage: Clearance of foreign materials via cilia and mucous in the nose, trachea, and/or bronchi.

mucositis: Inflammation of mucous membranes in the digestive tract, often as a side effect of chemotherapy or radiation.

nasogastric feeding tube: Feeding tube that travels from the nasal cavity through the pharynx to the stomach by way of the esophagus to meet short-term nutritional needs in patients with dysphagia.

neck breather: A person who, following a tracheotomy or total laryngectomy, breathes through a hole in the neck called a stoma.

neck dissection: Surgical procedure in which lymph nodes in the neck, affected by cancer, are removed.

necrosis: Death of body tissue.

nil per os (NPO): Status indicating that a patient is not to have any food orally, typically because of suspected or confirmed unsafe swallowing function.

nociceptive: Relating to pain that arises from the stimulation of nerve cells.

obturator: Small device that provides a smooth, rounded surface for guiding the insertion and removal of a tracheostomy tube.

occult: When referring to the cervical lymph nodes, indicative of microscopic metastasis that is not visible or palpable.

odynophagia: Painful swallowing.

oncology: Medical practice that focuses on the diagnosis and treatment of cancer.

oncology nurse: Nurse who specializes in the care of patients with cancer.

osteoradionecrosis: Bone death caused by radiation near the head or neck.

otolaryngologist: Physician who specializes in the medical and surgical treatment and management of conditions of the ear, nose, and throat (ENT) and related structures of the head and neck.

outer cannula: Main body of a tracheostomy tube that functions to keep an artificial airway in place and may be secured to the neck externally.

palliative care physician: Physician with specialized training in the management of physical and emotional pain or debilitating symptoms of chronic or serious illnesses such as cancer.

palliative medicine: Continuum of care that focuses on symptom and pain management (rather than cancer-directed curative treatment, which is the responsibility of other types of medical professionals) for patients with chronic or terminal disease.

partial laryngectomy: Surgical procedure to remove a portion of the larynx. *See* hemilaryngectomy laryngectomy, supraglottic laryngectomy, and supracricoid laryngectomy for details about specific types of partial laryngectomies.

pathologist: Physician with specialized training in studying cells or tissues to provide a definitive diagnosis for conditions such as cancer.

penetration: Occurs when food or liquid enters the larynx at the level of the vocal folds but does not pass below them.

pharyngeal stasis: Residue in the pharyngeal cavity during swallowing.

pharyngocutaneous fistula: Connection between the pharynx and cervical skin around a surgical incision site that may delay the initiation of oral food intake.

pharyngoesophageal segment: Band of muscular tissue the forms a transitional region between the pharynx and esophagus and is forced into vibration to enable tracheoesophageal and esophageal speech.

pneumatic artificial larynx: Artificial larynx that uses air from the tracheostoma to activate a vibratory response from human tissue, a metal or plastic reed, or a rubber membrane.

positron emission tomography (PET) scan: Type of diagnostic imaging that involves viewing dyed radioactive tracers that have been injected into the body to detect complex disease processes such as cancer.

primary care physician (PCP): Physician who serves as a patient's doctor for routine medical care and typically makes referrals to other specialists to manage complex medical issues such as laryngeal cancer.

pseudoepiglottis: Anatomic abnormality that often results after total laryngectomy in which a band of scar tissue, extending from the lateral pharyngeal wall to the base of the tongue, forms a small patch or pocket in which food or liquid may collect.

psychiatric-mental health nurse (PMHN): Nurse with specialized training and experience in assessing, diagnosing, and treating mental health conditions.

psychiatrist: Physician who diagnoses and treats psychological conditions, often by prescribing medication.

psychosocial oncology counselor: Medical professional who has extensive training in supporting patients with cancer who experience mental health concerns as part of their diagnosis or treatment processes.

radiation: Use of radioactive waves or rays externally or internally to kill cancer cells and prevent metastasis.

radiation oncologist: Physician who identifies the type and dosage of radiation treatment for patients with cancer.

respiratory therapist: Allied health professional who assists patients with breathing issues that result from diseases such as asthma, emphysema, or cancer.

rigid fiberoptic laryngoscopy: Examination that uses a rigid lighted endoscope that is inserted into the mouth and angled just over the base of a patient's tongue to visualize the larynx and vocal fold vibration during phonation on a sustained "ee" vowel.

saline bullet: Small vial of sterile saline used to provide temporary moisture to the airway via the stoma site in patients after tracheotomy or laryngectomy.

salvage partial (conservation) laryngectomy: Partial laryngectomy that occurs as a secondary measure after the failure of medical treatment (e.g., radiation or chemotherapy) for laryngeal cancer.

salvage surgery: Procedure performed to resect a tumor that has recurred after the failure of a primary treatment (i.e., radiation or chemotherapy).

salvage total laryngectomy: Total laryngectomy that occurs as a secondary measure after the failure of medical treatment (e.g., radiation or chemotherapy) for laryngeal cancer.

silent aspiration: Aspiration that occurs without any attempt to clear food or liquids that have passed into the airway.

sloughing: Separation of dead tissue from living tissue.

social worker: Allied health professional who facilitates the coordination of patient care and provides supportive services (e.g., counseling) for patients.

speaking valve: Device placed at the opening of a tracheostoma, at the neck, that allows exhaled air to flow through the vocal folds, mouth, and nose rather than directly through the stoma site.

speech: Verbal means of communication that occurs via the articulation of voiced or unvoiced sounds.

speech-language pathologist (SLP): Specialist in the diagnosis and treatment of speech, language, swallowing, and cognitive disorders across the lifespan.

staging of laryngeal cancer: Specialized process by which a laryngeal tumor is assigned a stage ranging from I (least advanced) to IV (most advanced) on the basis of its location, spread, and size; a cancer's stage facilitates predictions related to cure and/or response to treatment.

stoma: Temporary or permanent incision created in the trachea to enable respiration by way of the neck.

subglottic/subglottis: Area inferior to (below) the glottis. Subglottic is a term used to describe the location of structures, lesions, and/or food material in this region.

supracricoid laryngectomy: Sometimes called cricohyoidopexy or cricohyoidoepiglottopexy, this type of partial laryngectomy includes resection of the entire thyroid cartilage, true vocal folds, and paralaryngeal spaces with preservation of the cricoid cartilage and at least one arytenoid. The epiglottis is preserved in some cases and resected in others.

supraglottic laryngectomy: Type of partial laryngectomy in which structures above the level of the vocal folds are resected.

supraglottic/supraglottis: Area superior to (above) the glottis. Supraglottic is a term used to describe the location of structures, lesions, and/or food material in this region.

tissue resection: Surgical removal of all or part of a tissue.

total laryngectomy: Complete surgical removal of the larynx.

toxicity: Adverse side effects from cancer treatment, such as chemotherapy or radiation, on anatomical and physiological functioning.

trachea: Cartilaginous tube that connects the larynx to the lungs and allows for air inhaled at the mouth or nose to pass into the lower airway.

tracheoesophageal puncture (TEP): Surgically created fistula made in the back of the stoma site between the trachea and esophagus after laryngectomy to allow for the placement of a one-way prosthetic valve that facilitates tracheoesophageal speech.

tracheoesophageal speech: Form of alaryngeal speech in which a voice prosthesis, placed in a tracheoesophageal puncture site, enables air from the lungs to pass into the esophagus and vibrate the pharyngoesophageal segment.

tracheostoma: *See* stoma.

tracheostomy mask: Device designed to protect and administer oxygen at the site of a stoma.

tracheostomy tube: Tube that is placed in the trachea after tracheotomy surgery.

tracheotomy: Surgery that involves cutting through the neck and trachea to create an opening, called a stoma, in which a breathing tube (tracheostomy tube) can be inserted to create an airway.

videofluoroscopic swallowing study (VFSS): Examination that involves viewing swallowing function, via radiographic imaging, during the ingestion of various liquids and solids coated with barium.

vocal folds: Two bands of tissue that vibrate together to produce phonation, open to allow air to enter the lungs, and close to protect the airway.

voice: Sound produced via expiration of air through vibrating vocal folds.

voice prosthesis: Enables the generation of tracheoesophageal speech, prevents aspiration, and maintains a tracheoesophageal puncture site.

xerostomia: Dry mouth or a decrease in saliva.

Financial Disclosures

Julia R. Brennan has no financial or proprietary interest in the materials presented herein.

Lisa Crujido has no financial or proprietary interest in the materials presented herein.

Dr. Philip C. Doyle has no financial or proprietary interest in the materials presented herein.

Dr. Katharine E. Duckworth has no financial or proprietary interest in the materials presented herein.

Dr. Amy E. Engelhoven has no financial or proprietary interest in the materials presented herein.

Dr. Jennifer Campion Friberg has no financial or proprietary interest in the materials presented herein.

Tessa Goldsmith has no financial or proprietary interest in the materials presented herein.

Dr. Edie R. Hapner has no financial or proprietary interest in the materials presented herein.

Connor W. Hoban has no financial or proprietary interest in the materials presented herein.

Rachael E. Kammer has no financial or proprietary interest in the materials presented herein.

Dr. Richard P. McQuellon has not disclosed any relevant financial relationships.

Dr. Andrew J. Rosko has no financial or proprietary interest in the materials presented herein.

Dr. Andrew G. Shuman has no financial or proprietary interest in the materials presented herein.

Bonnie K. Slavych has no financial or proprietary interest in the materials presented herein.

Dr. Paul L. Swiecicki has no financial or proprietary interest in the materials presented herein.

Dr. Lisa A. Vinney has not disclosed any relevant financial relationships.

Index

Printed in the United States
by Baker & Taylor Publisher Services